Full Moon at Noontide

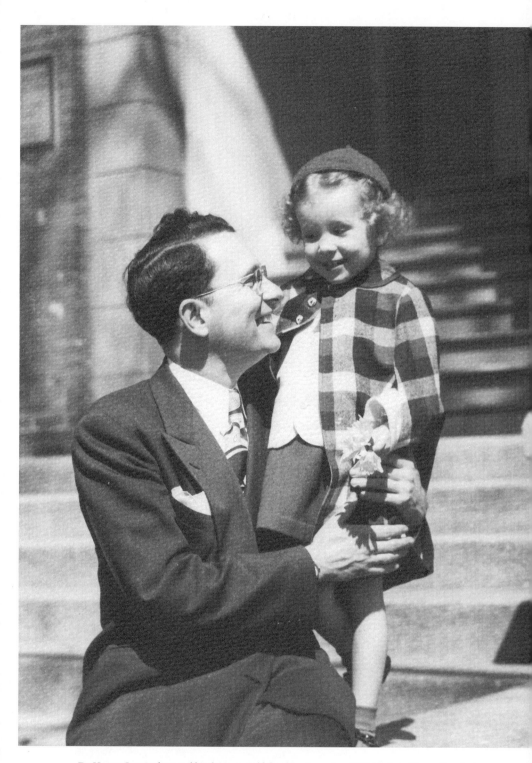

Dr. Homer Cunningham and his three-year-old daughter, Ann, circa 1949. Photo by Henry Cunningham

Full Moon at Noontide

A DAUGHTER'S LAST GOODBYE

Ann Putnam

Foreword by David Hilfiker, M.D.
Introduction by Thomas R. Cole

Medical Humanities
Thomas Mayo, series editor

SOUTHERN METHODIST
UNIVERSITY PRESS
Dallas

Requests for permission to reproduce material from this work should be sent to:
 Rights and Permissions
 Southern Methodist University Press
 PO Box 750415
 Dallas, Texas 75275-0415

Jacket and text design: Tom Dawson
Cover photograph: "Driftwood on New England Beach, circa 1950" by Dr. Homer Cunningham

Library of Congress Cataloging-in-Publication Data
 Putnam, Ann Lenore.
   Full moon at noontide : a daughter's last goodbye / Ann Putnam ; foreword by David
 Hilfiker ; introduction by Thomas R. Cole. — 1st ed.
     p. cm. — (Medical humanities)
   ISBN 978-0-87074-555-3 (alk. paper)
   1. Aging parents—Death—Psychological aspects. 2. Uncles—Death—Psychological aspects.
 3. Cunningham family. 4. Putnam, Ann Lenore—Family. 5. Putnam, Ann Lenore—Biography.
 6. College teachers—Washington (State)—Biography. 7. Women college teachers—Washington
 (State)—Biography. 8. Adult children of aging parents—Washington (State)—Biography.
 9. Cunningham, Grace, 1915-2006—Last years. 10. Cunningham, Henry—Last years. 11.
 Cunningham, Homer F.—Last years. I. Title. II. Series: Medical humanities.
   HQ1073.5.U62W37 2009
   155.9'370922—dc22
   [B]

                                                                    2009018023

Printed in the United States of America on acid-free paper

10   9   8   7   6   5   4   3   2   1

To Ed

"We need to be each others' storytellers—at least we have to try. . . .
Still, it is like painting the sky. What stars have been left out . . . ? But it
is a fearful task, each telling of the great tale. The night is dark.
I hear the wind pacing. . . . I feel the heart, at the door of its body,
going down the long stone stairs and out of this world, alone."

Mary Oliver, from *Blue Pastures*

Contents

Foreword

The journey into infirmity, old age, and death is rarely described both honestly and beautifully. It is not, after all, a pleasant trip; most of us are rightfully afraid of it—if not of death itself, certainly of infirmity and old age. And so we elide over the shame-inducing details—"the missed step, the crumbs down the front of the blouse, the stains on the tie, the unbrushed hair, the button missed, the zipper undone, the dentures soaking in a glass on the sink"—because we see ourselves somehow managing to avoid them. Our individual fantasies may be different. My father wanted to go suddenly from health to death, and a heart attack gave him his wish; he missed the most difficult parts of infirmity and old age. I imagine myself with a lingering final illness, moving quickly through the five stages of dying to acceptance, perched in my deathbed saying long goodbyes and offering grieving friends and family consolation. But most of us, perhaps unconsciously, fear the indignity. In *Full Moon at Noontide* Ann Putnam offers us the gift of a loving look . . . at the full catastrophe. "A thing whole and complete has a beauty of its own, even when the things apart are too terrible to say," she writes and then weaves the complex parts of the deaths of her father, mother, and uncle into something whole and complete and beautiful.

As a young doctor living in Grand Marais, Minnesota, I visited our small town's nursing home once a month, as per Medicare regulations, to see the ten or fifteen patients under my care. Since the nursing home staff generally cared well for my patients, and emergencies were treated as they arose, there usually wasn't much technical medical work to do on my monthly rounds, so I spent most of the morning just visiting, listening to the men and women as they told me about their lives. Some, like Paul Berglund, seemed to be shining lights of resilience— always ready to smile, always grateful. Paul had as many problems as the next person—including an intermittently painful abdominal aortic aneurysm—but he always seemed to see the bright side. The nurse said he was always like that.

Then there was Matt Hill, a lumberjack from Finland in his late eighties. He'd come to the United States as a young man but had always worked in logging camps with other Finns, going to town once a week only to get drunk, so he knew little English. One by one his Finnish-speaking friends from the lumber camps had died or left town, so, outside of my Finnish wife's monthly visit, he never received visitors. So Matt was utterly alone all day, day after day, unable to communicate with anyone. What is it like to be old, alone, and incommunicado? Yet even he seemed cheerful and, according to my wife, reluctant to burden others with his sorrow. I was in my thirties at the time, and I liked to imagine that I would be like Paul or Matt as I aged.

But even then, I suspected I'd be more like Arnie Helgeson.

Arnie was always cranky, always complaining about something. The medication I'd given him for his pain in the knees didn't work, the food was bad, the nurses were uncaring, his family wouldn't visit, his roommate was too loud. On each visit, somehow, he always happened to be in a foul mood. He was old, his knees hurt, this was his last stop, and nobody seemed very happy to see him either. What would I be like in his place? I guessed I might hide it a little better, but I'd succumb to the pain, depression, and foul mood too.

Few of us recognize in advance how solitary are the journeys into infirmity, into old age, and into death. Few of us make preparations that actually prepare us. In our occasional visions of that future, we are usually accompanied by a loved one or friend who at least understands. It's only when we get there that we realize it's always a journey into a never-before-explored land and that—regardless of who is near and how much they love us—we are finally alone in uncharted territory. We may be surprised to find that other people—even those who love us— have only limited interest in the particulars of our difficult exploration. While our pain, our weakness, our sexual dysfunction, our loneliness, our depression, our loss of balance and coordination take great personal courage to face, they are not terribly interesting topics of conversation to anyone else, and we will be truly solitary explorers. As Ann Putnam writes of herself confronted by her parents' aging: "I was not ready to hear of the ravages and insults of old age. I could not bear this then, not the details of that road awaiting us all." It's always an uncertain time, full of unexpected surprises, sometimes with opportunities for great heroism, no less heroic for being largely unrecognized.

Frequently there is little opportunity to adjust to one loss before another hits. Some of us, I'm sure, imagine some of our losses ahead of time. But we rarely count on the fact that some of the losses will be of the faculties we use to deal with losses. We may not think as well. We have less tolerance. We are more emotionally labile.

And we know it's not going to get better.

All this sounds, of course, depressing. And from many angles, it is depressing. But, "a thing whole and complete has a beauty of its own, even when the things apart are too terrible to say." In this memoir you are about to read, Ann Putnam brings you as close as you will probably get before it's your own turn to experience that journey into old age, infirmity, and death. The story appears to be a straightforward account of the last several years in the life of three old people: a long-married couple and the husband's twin brother. It's filled with what you might expect: strokes, cancer, dementia, and all the indignities of getting old and dying. But this is more a story than a memoir, more "a casting of raw, bitter facts into arcs of light." It is a poem that reveals the shimmering thin place between the "normal" world to which we're accustomed and the world to which we will journey.

Joseph's House in Washington, D.C., is a home, community, and hospice for previously homeless men and women with AIDS and/or cancer. Our family lived there for three years after its founding, and I have worked there for most of the last eighteen years. While there are certainly important exceptions, few of our residents have a daughter like Ann Putnam who is seeking to find the interstices between her world and theirs; they don't have a family eager to accompany them or love them unconditionally; they don't have personal pasts full of worldly accomplishments of which they can be proud. And so they must confront their infirmity and death without a net, without any of the usual supports.

Sometimes it's an unremittingly agonizing process: physical pain, shame, denial, loneliness, distrust, fear. Staff members do all they can to welcome the new resident, to ameliorate the pain, to provide a nonjudgmental, accepting presence, to love them; yet often the resident cannot accept our caring and dies in his or her pain, denial, and isolation.

But sometimes the transformation is near to miraculous. As a resident moves closer to the thin place, he becomes peaceful and accepting; he accepts not only the ministrations of the staff but the staff members themselves. Racial and class differences melt away; the injustice that was so frequently responsible for his illness and death is forgiven. Dying and death is accompanied by much love and is, yes, beautiful.

What is consistently awe-inspiring to me is the transformation of the staff at Joseph's House. Every year we welcome three to five interns who spend a low-paid, essentially volunteer year with us. Most are recent college graduates doing a year of service before moving on to the next phase of their lives. A few are older and much more experienced. All of them come to this place of dying with anxiety and fear. They are usually white and affluent; the residents are almost all black and poor. One marker of staff members' anxiety is their discomfort at spending time just sitting there with a dying person. Frequently there is little to *do*. Sure, medications must be intermittently given, bed clothes changed, bodies bathed, and so on. But mostly the task is just to *be* there, doing nothing, usually not even saying anything. For most people at first, it's not easy.

Over the course of the volunteer's year with us, however, something changes dramatically. Accompaniment is still sometimes difficult—especially if the resident is in pain or otherwise uncomfortable. But the *being there* becomes increasingly a gift—both for the dying resident and for the volunteer. The thin place between the everyday world and whatever is next becomes more real and more beautiful; it becomes, if anything, even thinner, and the volunteers sense the deep privilege of being there. For most volunteers the experience is profoundly transformational. They have, it seems to me, seen and accompanied the souls of others and have experienced the essential unity of human beings. "We are all one" is now more than a philosophic or theological position; it is now for them an experienced reality.

These things are difficult to express well in the medium of essay that is only rational; rather, the metaphors and rhythms of story and poetry are necessary to pull back the curtain on this numinous other world for us. *Full Moon at Noontide* is such a story.

David Hilfiker

David Hilfiker, M.D., is the founder of Joseph's House in Washington, D.C., a community for homeless men and women with AIDS. He is the author of *Urban Injustice: How Ghettos Happen, Not All of Us Are Saints: A Doctor's Journey with the Poor*, and *Healing the Wounds: A Doctor Looks at His Work*.

Introduction

Despite Hobbes's pessimistic claim that life is "nasty, brutish, and short," people everywhere and always have wanted to live a long and healthy life. In fact, the entire project of Western scientific medicine has been motivated by the dream of long life. And in the latter half of the twentieth century, this dream was realized in Western developed countries. Most of our citizens live well into their seventies and eighties, and many into their nineties. Even some of the chronic diseases of old age are in retreat. Advances in science and technology, along with improved strategies of self-care, continue to yield more years free of disability.

There is no precedent in human history for our era of mass longevity. On the one hand, this new abundance of healthy life is a gift that we are not quite sure how to open. And on the other hand, we do not know how to live well in the face of those traditionally intractable elements of aging—decline and death. Consumer culture sells us the image of growing old without aging. But despite the hype of "anti-aging" medicine and the advertisements of drug companies and assisted living facilities, we have postponed rather than vanquished frailty, disease, disability, and mortality. Granted, there are some scientists and physicians who view aging as a disease that will eventually be cured. But most scientists, geriatricians, and policymakers have a more modest goal—to preserve function and delay the onset of disability until close to the time of a person's death. In this scenario, older people would die pretty much in the manner of Oliver Wendell Holmes's "One-Hoss Shay" (horse carriage), which fell apart "all at once and nothing first." Sadly, only 20 percent of us will die this way—after a short period of decline, with rapid deterioration limited to the final weeks and days before death. Another 20 percent of us will die after several years of increasing physical limitation, punctuated by acute life-threatening episodes requiring hospitalization and medical intervention. And 40 percent of us will die after a prolonged period (perhaps even a decade) of decline due to dementia, stroke, or the frailty of several body systems.

"All things toil to weariness," we read in Ecclesiastes. "Man cannot utter it." No one wants to feel or endure the pain and suffering of elders and family members caught in the downward spiral of physical decline. It is unspeakable. We collude in a conspiracy to suppress, avoid, and disguise the misery. So we need our writers, artists, and poets to utter the unutterable, to put the mirror of truth before our eyes, to reveal what T. S. Eliot described as "the cold friction of expiring sense." If we can bear it, our artists (like our religious leaders) help us face the things we are most afraid of and show us that we can rise to the occasion—even catch glimpses of the sacred in the darkest times.

I received the manuscript of Ann Putnam's memoir, *Full Moon at Noontide: A Daughter's Last Goodbye*, one month after my ninety-one-year-old mother-in-law died in Dallas. For years, she had lain in bed incapacitated, receiving extraordinary round-the-clock care. She could not get out of bed, could barely speak, and only swallowed with great difficulty while someone was spoon-feeding her. With great courage and dignity, she endured constant and wrenching coughs, as her body tried to dislodge food that passed into her lungs instead of her stomach. Yet her great wit and will never failed her, and she was nurtured by the love of her family and caregivers. In her last year, the family traveled to Dallas during multiple hospitalizations; from each she emerged weaker than before. A feeding tube was out of the question. In the last week of her life, she struggled terribly for breath. "I don't want to do this anymore," she told her loving caregiver. Hospice was called. Small doses of morphine eased her breathing, and we gathered for an agonizing death vigil. When she died, no one was comforted by the fact that she had lived a long and full life. On the contrary: the longer the life, the greater the loss.

When SMU editor Kathryn Lang asked if I would write a brief essay for Ann Putnam's memoir, I saw my mother-in-law lying on her deathbed, breathing tenaciously against all predictions, hovering between this world and the next. I was haunted by those exhausting nights when we stood around her bed for hours, wondering when she would breathe her last breath. Still sleepwalking in that heavy, grief-laden fog that somehow helps us cope with what we cannot accept or understand, I didn't feel ready to open my heart to another person's experience of losing her parents. In spite of myself, I told Kathryn I'd read the manuscript. I googled Ann Putnam and learned that she is a novelist and professor of English at the University of Puget Sound. I thought about the recent spate of caregiver stories, which however heartfelt, never rise to the level of literature. As I often do with longer texts, I started reading Putnam's memoir on a plane ride from Houston to New York, thinking I'd breeze through it and write Kathryn a quick note saying that I was too busy.

From the beginning, *Full Moon at Noontide* seduced me. Then it sliced me open, slapped me in the face, made me cry, and enlarged my spirit. The memoir tells the story of the elders in Putnam's family—the slow decline and death of her father, her mother, and her father's bachelor twin brother. It begins with her father's stroke at age eighty-two—Homer Cunningham, a retired professor of history living in Spokane with his wife and his brother. Two years earlier, at age eighty, he had looked and acted like a man of sixty-five.

"Doesn't it always begin that way?" Putnam writes. "A telephone call across the miles, one reality exchanged for another in an instant. Not that you weren't waiting for it all along in some dark place of your mind where you hold such things that cannot yet be brought into the light."

Immediately, she looks for escape routes. This must be a dream, she thinks. Or, it should have happened *this* way. (What *really* happened was that her father languished in the emergency room for three hours and missed the window of time when the clot could have been dissolved.) Then, she looks for consolation: "I wondered if there were laws of compensation for such things, if something came in its place. Something simpler, purer, a distillation of spirit after all." Or maybe things can be fixed through faith: "I want to exorcise that brain clot, restore the damaged connections, fill in the blank spaces with love." Not only does Putnam lose her parents and uncle over the course of two years but her husband also dies of cancer just three months before she finishes the manuscript, and we are left wondering how it is possible to survive such heartbreak.

In her ongoing struggle against meaninglessness and despair, Putnam deploys the weapons of her craft—language, narrative, and metaphor. From Thoreau, she learned early that "brutal facts [can] flower into understanding." Can the right language somehow redeem her suffering, or his? Briefly, she lets us inside the intolerable wrestling with words and images: ". . . oh how I have searched for the metaphor for what happened to my father. I want to gather it all up into a constellation of meaning so that he was not just some old guy dragging an arm and a leg through what life remained to him."

Stories, my friend Marc Kaminsky says, are "mortal oars for rowing across the wide waters of oblivion to make the round trips toward meaning." Or to borrow a different metaphor from Kenneth Burke, stories are "equipment for living." They keep our ancestors alive and link one generation to another. Putnam's Uncle Henry, for example, was such a difficult man that her children told outrageous stories to make it bearable to be around him. "They were stories that could save our love from the erosion that his old age exacted upon him and upon us. What is a story anyway, but a casting of raw, bitter facts into arcs of light?"

Writing autobiographical and family stories is perilous work, filled with difficult decisions about what to leave in and what to remove, what to reveal, what to conceal, and whose feelings may be hurt. Sometimes, for the sake of the story, one violates confidentiality or other promises. Putnam decided to reveal certain family secrets and to include her mother in the narrative, even though she had promised otherwise. She shares some of these difficult decisions and other vulnerabilities with her readers, and we trust her for it. But it is the profound love for her family that animates all the craft and wins our hearts. We stay with the story because it is so beautifully written, because it is ultimately our story as well, and because Putnam shows us that love—not death—can have the last word.

For all its pain and perils, the work of writing stories is also a means of healing, of recovering and getting one's bearings at new junctures on the journey of life. Along with our gratitude and admiration for this deep and powerful memoir, we can only hope that Putnam's long loving labor has brought her a measure of peacefulness and hope for the future.

Thomas R. Cole

Thomas R. Cole is director of the McGovern Center for Health, Humanities, and the Human Spirit at the University of Texas–Houston Health Science Center Medical School. The author of many books on aging, including *The Journey of Life: A Cultural History of Aging in America*, he is also a professor of humanities and religious studies at Rice University.

Preface

This is the story of my mother and father and my dashing, bachelor uncle, my father's identical twin, and how they lived together with their courage and their stumblings, as they made their way into old age and then into death. And it's the story of the journey from one twin's death to the other, of what happened along the way, of what it means to lose the other who is also oneself.

My story takes the reader through the journey of the end of life: selling the family home, relocation at a retirement community, doctor's visits, ER visits, specialists, hospitalizations, ICUs, nursing homes, hospice. It takes the reader through the gauntlet of the health care system with all the attendant comedies and sorrows, joys and terrors of such things. Finally it asks: What consolation is there in growing old, in such loss? What abides beyond the telling of my own tale? Wisdom carried from the end of the journey to readers who are perhaps only beginning theirs. Still, what interest might there be in reading of this inevitable journey taken by such ordinary people? Turned to the light just so, the beauty and laughter of the telling transcend the darkness of the tale.

During the final revisions of this book, my husband was dying of cancer, and he died before I could finish it. What I know so far is this: how pure love becomes when it is distilled through such suffering and loss—a blue flame that flickers and pulses in the deepest heart.

As I finish this book he is gone three months.

Full Moon at Noontide

Lights Go Out

When did it all begin? That long, slow descent into the last good-night, that sweet, sad goodbye, knit up of so many small good-byes. Goodbye to the right hand, goodbye to the right leg, goodbye to dialing the phone, or knowing what day or time it is, or wanting to eat, or remembering to swallow—but never goodbye to knowing who we were.

It's a Friday and the Seattle late-afternoon traffic is already piling up, though as soon as I can shift into the express lanes it will be smooth sailing home. But it's always a perilous turn into those lanes that rush through the dark tunnel under the freeway.

When I make the turn, suddenly there is my father before me. He takes a step, then falls to the side and crumples to the floor—not in my mind's eye or memory but from someplace outside myself, an image that comes unmoored from its holdings across the miles and floats across my face. It lasts only seconds, just a flicker, barely a vision, but something turns over in me. I flick on my lights, pay extra attention. The traffic suddenly feels treacherous, cars shifting lanes precipitously, a car horn echoing long and mournfully inside that expressway tunnel. It's dark for way too long. I want to be back in the light because I know that three hundred miles away in Spokane something has happened that will change everything. Some way I know that losing him has begun in earnest. It's Friday, the thirteenth of September, 1997.

Not that I haven't suspected something like this for several years now. So many things already gone wrong, like the mysterious bone marrow failure, and then the usual laundry list of getting old—diabetes, high blood pressure. Still, he has a lovely vitality, a buoyancy, a good and kind spirit that greets the world with promise and laughter. Always rushing off to the Whitworth College campus, where he'd taught so many years, to take photographs or to attend political meetings across town or to his Monday date with Rotary.

The winter before, back home in Spokane for Christmas, I take a snowy walk with my father. We go a block or two, then he shrugs off for home. It's near midnight and the snow is falling all around, and I can see his face in the streetlight. "I just can't do this like I used to. I'm sorry," he says. We are across the street from the house now, and he turns to head on in, then looks back at me. "I've got to get your mother someplace safe." He looks weary, a little frightened. "I don't know what's going to happen to me."

"Dad," I say, "what are you talking about?" Of course I know. That bone marrow failure they're saying could turn into a slow-growing leukemia that's shadowed him for over a year now.

"We need someplace to go," he says. "This house is too much for us." We both look across the street at that three-story house, the yard, the driveway, the roof, all covered in snow. He wants me to find a retirement community for them where there is no snow to shovel, no icy sidewalks, no stairs to fall down, somewhere in Seattle near where my husband and I live. My father is eighty-two.

"Okay," I say to him.

"I never thought I'd get old," he says, shaking his head.

I give him a hug. "It's okay, Dad. Everything's gonna be okay."

"I love you, Pill," he says, invoking my childhood nickname. "Don't go much farther. It's too late to be out here by yourself." I stand there watching him making his perilous way across the street, how he holds the railing as he goes up the stairs to the front porch. There is snow on his shoulders, his scarf, his cap. He stamps his feet and goes inside. Tears run down my face. I look up at the heavy gray sky. It's snowing furiously now, and so I turn in too. No sense in walking out here alone.

Then I'm out of the tunnel and into the light laying itself on the waters of Lake Union busy with sailboats out for an early-evening sail. The skyline is blazing with sunset. I glance back at the Space Needle behind me in fast-falling light. The Olympic Mountains are purple now in the hastening twilight, and suddenly I know I need to get on home.

It's the second weekend in September, and Courtney, my daughter, who starts back to college on Monday, is waiting for me at home. We're celebrating with tickets for the Gypsy Kings. My husband, Ed, is off in the Straits on an end-of-summer fishing trip with his best buddy, who's the only one he knows who loves fishing as much he does. When I drive up the hill I see her watching out the window for me. She doesn't do jumping jacks or send me a clownish wave, like always. She's just standing there in the middle of the living room.

"What's wrong?" I say, as I come inside, reading the shorthand in her eyes.

"Grandpa had a stroke," she says with no preamble, and no way to soften it.

Doesn't it always begin that way? A telephone call across the miles, one reality exchanged for another in an instant. Not that you weren't waiting for it all along in some dark place of your mind where you hold such things that cannot yet be brought into the light. You wish for a bad connection, crossed lines, a lapse in hearing, a rush into dream. But you're only hearing what you fear, though none of it seems real.

I call my mother. She's as stoic and noncommittal as ever. No need to rush across the state right now, no danger anymore. He'll be moved to rehab in a few days. But I can sense the fear in her voice. When I ask to talk to him, she says not right now. This alarms me more than anything. Tomorrow, she says. I think she's afraid he might cry into the phone.

Then I wonder if it's because his brain is scrambled, if his speech is gone. But she can read my mind. She knows where I'm headed. "Just a weakness on the right side," she says, understated as always. What she doesn't say of course is *crippled*. Half of him is useless now. She tells me he'll get better, that he'll be moved to rehab where they will bring the right side of him back to life. As if half of him is just off somewhere taking a nap, and only needs a good, stiff shake. But I want to hear his voice. I want to know that he's really there, that he is himself.

She tells me how they were just sitting in their chairs reading the newspaper after breakfast. My father goes to get up and slips out of the chair and slumps onto the floor. No prelude, no fanfare, nothing like that firebrand rushing up your left arm, no elephant on your chest—just a soft, quiet, slipping down. "Grace, I can't get up!" he says to my mother in such surprise she drops her newspaper and rushes to kneel beside him, while she scoops up the phone, as if she's been practicing this gesture for years. My uncle, who lives with them now, is downstairs in his room sleeping in.

This is how it *should* have happened: After the rush to the ER, an angel of a doctor comes in with an IV and plugs him into a miracle drug that brings to life what he thought had died—the arm and leg asleep by his side, the mouth shaped in a cry that never comes, the sounds he makes we do not understand, thoughts he will never have again. It's only a matter of days before he is himself again. And all the terrors that might have been have gone around some bend in the road for good.

But this is how it *really* happened: Three hours later—and that's all the time they've got before that clot's dark surprise cannot be undone—and they still haven't begun to dissolve it. They have not rushed him for an MRI or CAT scan to see what kind of stroke it is. That magical three-hour window of opportunity has come and gone. No miracle doctor, no miracle cure. Then it's too late for anything that can stop the brain death going on just out of reach. "They didn't do anything for me. They just let me lie there," my anguished father says. They just let him disappear into the glacial pace of any ER. I wondered then as now if they had not rushed to treat him because they thought he was just a throwaway old man.

I was told later there is some risk to this miracle drug, and it's true: things may have been more complicated in reality than they seemed over the phone. But it was a choice my father never got to make: Take this treatment and you're cured. You can walk out of here as before. On the other hand, this treatment might kill you. It's up to you, old man. Which way do you want it? He'd have chosen life. He'd have reached out for the brass ring and risked losing his balance completely. And my mother? I know what my mother would have chosen. She would not have abided the risk. She would kept as much of him safe as she could. Well, it would have been a house divided.

Because my mother did not call me at school, I had no vote, not that it was mine to give. She waited until I'd finished my teaching day and was on the long commute home before she called. "What could you have done?" she'd said later. If I'd been in that ER I would have run into the hallway and grabbed the first white coat I saw and screamed, don't just let him *lie* there. For God's sake *do* something. I would have remembered that magic potion and shouted its name. I'd had that bit of information tucked away somewhere for safekeeping for a long time now. But if she'd managed to reach me at school, I would have whispered its name fiercely over the phone. And later, I would have tentatively asked her—"Did Dad ever get that t-PA?"—because either he did or he didn't, and by now it was far too late for that.

Ah, the stroke. Grandpa had a stroke. Such a bitter cliché. Can't walk straight, talk straight, think straight. He's just leftovers now. A stroke is obscene. It twists the smile of your face, one side can't laugh or cry, speech is a tape come unwound, you mean one thing and say another, you laugh when you should cry, the right arm flops at your side, the right leg drags across the floor, everything tilts to the right, weighted forever to earth. And the mind. The precious mind. How it had reasoned things out all those years, put things together, taken them apart, seen them new and whole again. Now suddenly up is down. Visible proof of all the little deaths inside.

Have a heart attack instead, if you could choose. A heart attack gets all the attention. After the initial heart-stopping pain, of course, and some residual weakness and shortness of breath and terrors you cannot name. Maybe a little paleness around the eyes, a slower step going up the stairs, the cheekbones at a sharper angle, but only in a certain light, and who couldn't afford to drop a few pounds anyway? Have a heart attack any day, if you could choose such things. A heart attack gets all that rushing about, the paddles ready for rescue if the heart monitor goes flat. I'd seen enough medical TV. A heart attack doesn't leave you on a gurney for three hours while your brain cells vanish into thin air.

I wondered what it would be like, this spreading darkness in the brain. A string of Christmas lights going out one by one. Plugs loose in their sockets. The right arm and leg not exactly numb, but detached from the will. Or body parts that look like yours but really belong to somebody else. Not that you'd mind missing an arm or leg, or a few words here and there, or a few thoughts you couldn't think anymore, so long as you lived. So long as the core of you remained, there was no reason to shout or call out. No reason to complain about the slow service in the ER.

Imagine waking up mornings unrecognizable to yourself. Like Gregor Samsa on that first morning of the metamorphosis. But wouldn't you permit yourself a few golden moments of forgetting, in order to remember life as it had been on some fine morning with the sun streaming in your window, and you ready to turn to your wife and touch her there and there and there?

I wondered if there were laws of compensation for such things, if something came in its place. Something simpler, purer, a distillation of spirit after all. Was it a worthy exchange for an arm and a leg?

That was Emerson. Or was it laws of correspondence? Emerson was never my guide anyway. It was always Thoreau, with his uncompromising, luminous facts. How he could believe in the miracle of Walden Pond and still have to know if it was truly bottomless as myth would have it. And then front the measurable fact that it wasn't. I loved the realism of Thoreau and the transcendence.

I loved Thoreau because of my father. It was my first term in graduate school at the University of Washington, and I was terrified I would not be good enough or smart enough, and any day they would find out it had been a mistake to let me in. And my first assignment in my first course: read Thoreau's *Journals*, all fourteen volumes of them, and write a paper about some progression you saw playing out as you read. A single set of journals on reserve in the library that could not be checked out, but had to be read in the library in two-hour stretches. It would take me months to read those journals sitting at a library table in the reserve room two hours at a time. I already had Courtney, my year-old baby, to take care of, and my two little boys, Chris and Robb. I couldn't read fourteen volumes of journals in the library and write a paper in three weeks.

I was in tears when I called him. My graduate school career would be over before it had even begun. I started to laugh then began to cry. All my life I had known that my father would do anything for me. And so it was. Some way he charmed the librarian at Whitworth College, where he was a professor of history, into letting him check out Thoreau's *Journals*, all fourteen volumes of them, on reserve in their library also. She was keen on him anyway, and believed everything Professor Homer Cunningham told her. But how he explained his intentions with the *Journals* I cannot imagine even now. I remember her as a pinched and suspicious woman who liked books best when they stayed on their shelves. These were rare or semirare books that were never, under any circumstance, to leave the reserve room of the library. It's a good thing she never knew that he was going to put them in cardboard boxes and take them to the bus station to make their way from Spokane to Seattle in the cargo hold of a Greyhound bus, for my own luxuriant use. When I got them home and unpacked them, I lined them up on the couch and took their picture.

And reading them I fell in love with rain, and the clouds moving across the sky, and the first green slips of spring you wouldn't notice unless you knew how to look and see that you had survived the hard season of winter once more. And that just as promised, there it was after all, joy in abundance. Plenitude after all. Those weeks with my very own Thoreau and the rain drumming on the skylight above where I read, the comfort of my abiding father kept me safe from all winter storms.

That semester I fell in love with Thoreau and his metaphors. The fact would always flower into significance for Thoreau. He only needed solitude and time. "I grew like corn in the night," he wrote in *Walden*. During his dreaming time the metaphor was born. But writing this now, I wonder if it is the same for me. Christmas lights, legs and arms unmoored, plugs and sockets. And later an ice storm, and other such metaphors down the line. Why not describe the behavior of damaged neurons instead and leave embellishments behind? Just measure the damned pond, not fabricate some dreaming symbol. But oh how I have searched for the metaphor for what happened to my father. I want to gather it all up into a constellation of meaning so that he was not just some old guy dragging an arm and a leg through what life remained to him. I would seek the metaphor I needed, the thing I could rub between my fingers, then tuck away in my pocket like a lucky charm. Metaphor would draw me close, not push me away. I would let the brutal facts flower into understanding. Maybe what I knew from memory and an imagination forged in love might, if I were so lucky, yield a greater truth that would extend beyond all the sorrows to come and my anguished part in them.

How does it feel to be turning eighty and look sixty-five? my father's internist had asked. And it was true. When I think of him even now I see the handsome wavy-haired man with the broad face and smile; the beckoning, interested, interesting eyes; the easy laugh; the suppleness of voice, emotion, thought. I can see him dashing out the door to his little Honda Civic to rush over to campus to the darkroom where he'd spend hours developing his historical photographs—or maybe see some students, check out a book or two, or maybe fourteen. So many projects, so many deadlines, always the last professor on campus to turn in his grades, until the registrar threatened to come to the house and snatch them up. No worries, she was keen on him too. And more than a decade into retirement, the same. Always on the go. Such happiness, such joy, every day a promise of all good things. Right up until that Friday morning when he slipped out of the chair and said my mother's name.

"Hi, Dad," I say the next day when I finally get him on the phone.

"Hi, Pill," my father says. "I had a stroke."

"I know," I say and start to add I'm sorry, but can't get the words out, so I just let the silence hang thick and mournful between us. I wish for something funny for either of us to say, like always. From now on I'll have to provide the comic relief for both of us, but I don't know that yet. Because one of the things that has disappeared is my father's ready sense of humor, his buoyant easy laugh, like bubbles rising in air, the way he would break into song in his rich tenor voice when a tune came into his head, or sometimes just a single note he could match from music on television or the radio, or the way he loved to answer the phone with "Duffy's Tavern." Gone. All gone.

"You're still my Pill," he says. He's always called me that because he said I was his pill for happiness. What he's really saying is that he's still himself. He's still my father. He's still in need of me.

Strangely, he doesn't sound that different over the phone. Only like a bad connection. His voice on the phone is a little subdued, croaky, as if his throat is dry, but his speech isn't garbled like I'd feared. My mother has told me how mentally intact he is. There cannot be enough gratitude for that. But I need to see him. I want to see his face. I want to put my arms around him, kiss his forehead, take his hand. It would be enough. He wouldn't even have to say anything. He could go in silence forever. My anger over the magic potion is gone. Now I'm like my mother. I wouldn't have him risk falling off the horse to grab that brass ring an inch or two out of reach.

I want to exorcise that brain clot, restore the damaged connections, fill in the blank places with love. Incantations, healing crystals, smoke and mirrors. I had already said a thousand prayers. I had almost lost him, and now I can't see him enough.

Then it's a week later and my husband and I and Alex, our eighty-five-pound Alaskan malamute, have all piled into the car and made the three-hundred-mile trek across the state. Since this isn't exactly an emergency, at least not yet, we don't pull the kids out of their college classes that have only just begun. For Chris and Robb and Courtney, the threesome, it's a reprieve.

We drive straight to the hospital and then there he is. He's sitting in a wheelchair, listing to the right, counting down the minutes until he can be put back to bed. Sitting in the wheelchair is part of his rehab now. He's looking up at the television or at my mother who sits in the blue vinyl chair in the corner, keeping watch. He's wearing his blue sweater, his beige khakis. I'm grateful there is no hospital gown and robe, no thin white blanket over his knees, no little hospital socks on his feet. No. He's all dressed for the day. Except for the fact that he can't sit up straight in his chair, except for the fact that it's a wheelchair, all looks as it was.

"Hi, Dad," I say.

"Oh my," my father says softly, shaking his head as I put my arms around him. "I'm so glad to see you." He starts to cry. "I'm sorry to be like this," he says. It's the first time I have ever seen him cry.

"It's okay, Dad. Everything's okay." He just looks at me. He has nothing to say because right now nothing is okay. Except that we have come, except that now he has seen my face, his only child's face.

And his face, his precious face, is no landscape of disaster. His speech is not altered. And he's thinking straight as far as we can tell. But of course it's the beginning of the end.

"I'm so tired," he says to my mother. He says his back is hurting, and no wonder, sitting slumped over to the right like that.

"We've been calling to get him back in bed," my mother says with an edge in her voice. "Everybody's busy, apparently." She's holding on tight. She's hunkered down for the long haul and is conserving every effort. My father doesn't trust the hospital staff yet, and I can see the fear in his eyes even his smile cannot hide. But soon, in his own fashion, they will all be wonderful, and he will become everybody's favorite patient. He'll work so hard to please everybody, to prove that he's still himself and the effort will exhaust him.

Then my husband says, "Okay, Dad," and leans over. "Put your arms around my neck. I've got you." And so he gathers him up out of the wheelchair and lays him down on top of the bed, puts a pillow under his knees. Even then I know this image will stay with me. My father in my husband's arms.

"Oh, that's better," he says. "Thank you, Ed."

What is an old man anyway? Someone grown more precious for the years, not less. Such an accumulation of memory and love. I look at my father exhausted from sitting in the chair then look over at the man in the bed next to him, who stares at the ceiling. He'll be gone the next week when we come back to visit. He will be dead and gone. The contrast between the two of them comforts me. My father has had his stroke and has made it safely to the other side.

We don't stay long. We take my mother home. She is also weary beyond speaking. She's been keeping watch all day. Alex, who has been in the car for six hours already, needs to get a walk.

My Uncle Henry, my father's identical twin, has been waiting by the phone in the house the three of them share, in case anything happens. But of course it has already happened, though he can imagine things far worse. My mother has banned him from coming to the hospital. He'd pace the floor outside my father's hospital room, carrying his fear in his hands like a sword, brandishing it at everyone he sees. He trusts no one to know what they're doing and tells them so. He is anguished to the core. His voice comes out high and shaky, and though he has tried mightily to hold on to himself, he cannot keep the terrors in check. It irritates my mother beyond bearing, though she knows what this is all about. He's in that bed too. What has happened to my father has also happened to him. Now he's trying to save his brother from the disasters he sees at every turn. The twins: Homer and Henry.

We sit in the TV room and catch my uncle up on the latest developments at the hospital, though there is nothing much to report. He's sitting in his TV chair, strangely silent, looking off across the room. My mother's in her chair; my husband and I are across the room on the couch. I look at my father's empty chair and know for the first time what a terrible thing has happened. The tears ache inside my head, gather in my throat. The dog sniffs my father's chair, then goes over to my mother and nudges her hand. Alex adores my father, though he does not quite reciprocate the devotion. And there is so much of her, this enormous dog, who insists on giving my father kisses he does not want. It's because she knows he doesn't love her like the rest of us do that she's still trying to win him over. My father and uncle did not grow up with animals. Their mother thought animals carried germs and fleas, and so were not allowed.

I look around the room. My silent mother, my uncle, who is acting as protector of the family while my father is laid up, the very image of my father but not my father. And my husband beside me. We just look at the TV, though none of us is really watching. I wish we had brought the children. They can always be counted on for comic relief. The dog is restless, can't figure out what's happening, keeps pacing through the house, looking out the front window, coming back to sniff my father's chair. She finally settles down in the corner, keeping watch.

"Is he any better?" my uncle finally brings himself to ask. He hasn't seen my father for a couple of days.

"Henry, it's going to take time," my mother snaps. "Don't keep *asking* me that."

"I'm sorry," he says. He' surprised at my mother's sharp tone, and oddly chastened. I wonder if he's thinking how his life will change, how maybe he'll be truly needed now. Not just an appendage, like before. Would he assume my father's place? I counted back. He'd lived with my parents for over twenty years, ever since his retirement from the Marshall, Michigan, School District, where he was an administrator, to take a job at Spokane Falls Community College teaching history and government.

Then too soon the weekend is over and Ed and I are heading for home back across the state. But we stop at the hospital for a last visit on our way out of town. We let Alex out for a last-minute walk around the parking lot. I lead her over to an attractive strip of grass, but she pulls the other way, hard, back across the parking lot toward the hospital. And she doesn't stop until the sliding doors snap open. Then she looks over her shoulder at us. I drop the leash just to see what she'll do, and she trots on in. I race in after her. She's standing in the lobby looking back at me. *Well, come on, let's go find him.* I grab her leash before someone can evict us. She's caught his scent on us, what he'd left behind, and figured out that he is in that place where we went without her. I wonder what else she knows. If she thinks he's in danger. There are many ways to know things, and I am only beginning to learn how many.

Of course, we might visit the hospital professionally, say as a pet therapy team. But she would have to undergo a personality transformation for that. She hates to be petted, thinks she's above all that. I know what she's thinking: I will always save you, but you don't have to pet me all the time. I have always loved her wildness, but she'd probably scare the little old ladies walking their IVs down the hall.

"We know there are some mental deficiencies. There have to be, given the location of his stroke," the doctors tell my mother. "We just haven't found them yet."

"They tested me and tested me and could find *nothing* wrong," my father says in anguish. "My mind is no different than it ever was." It's funny when he says it, and gives us a lead-in for any number of jokes. Dad, your mind was *always* different. But we hold them back. The mind is no cause for levity now. Ah, the mind. The PhD in history from NYU, the college professor, the politician, the photographer, the occasional fill-in preacher in those rural communities, favorite guest speaker, local Republican big shot, squiring congressmen, governors, and an occasional president around town. His mental faculties are intact, my mother repeats like a prayer. So we watch and guard against irresistible urges to see differences where we hope there are none. These mental acuity tests are the deepest indignity of all. They go far beyond the failures of the body. To question the integrity of the mind, after all, is the cruelest cut.

He's come to claim the stroke as his very own. Not *a* stroke, or even *the* stroke, but *my* stroke. Like my uncle announcing all these years: I'm having one of *my* sick headaches. My mother has always found it funny and curious—that possessiveness about some illnesses and not others. She'd say to me, "Well, you don't hear people talking about *my diarrhea*." But it's my mother's stroke too. You can see it in her face. She has forsaken her makeup, which she had always worn. It's not an oversight but seems more her pronouncement to the world that something has come to an end.

We're driving to Spokane almost every weekend now. On the fourth weekend, when my father's been in rehab for a month, he gets a weekend pass to go out for dinner. He's been there so long now he's afraid to leave the hospital, and they don't want him to become "institutionalized," as they call it. It takes all afternoon to get him ready for his first time out in the world. The first time out in the world in a wheelchair. But he's all dressed up in his camel blazer, brown wool pants, oxfords, shirt, and tie.

We drive into the parking lot to Shenanigans on the Spokane River, and pull into the handicapped space, with its blue outline of a wheelchair on the pavement. It's all still so new we don't have handicapped stickers yet, so my husband will get us safely into the restaurant and then move the car.

The lobby is crowded and Ed must edge the wheelchair between people heading in and out of the bar to the left. Some of them are carrying drinks to their table, or waiting with drinks in hand. My father looks up at them and hunches forward. All those drinks, all those people. It feels like a pub on St. Patrick's Day, but of course it's just a Saturday night in October. But there is some kind Oktoberfest celebration going on. Somebody bumps into the wheelchair and spills a little scotch or whiskey on my father's camel blazer. "Sorry," the man says quickly, and moves on. I want to rush after him and scream, "That's my *Dad* you just spilled your drink on." Then I realize from here on there will be all kinds of ways to fall to earth. We're in a different world, where the laws of gravity have taken on new meaning.

The hostess leads us to our table, and not until we get right to the edge of the three steps leading to the upper level do we remember our new place in the universe. We had forgotten to ask for handicapped seating. We can wait for another table in the crowded lobby, really almost a hallway, or we can wait a few minutes until they can improvise. Eventually they bring out a big piece of plywood that will serve as a ramp up which my husband negotiates the wheelchair. My father looks on with frightened eyes as he rises from one level to another. Such a wonder how things turn out. One minute you're sitting in your easy chair, reading the newspaper, and now you're being wheeled up a makeshift ramp in the middle of your favorite restaurant. It's a blessing not to notice the way people stare, then look away.

But then we're seated around a lovely table that looks out over the Spokane River shimmering in the late-afternoon sun. All that sunlight, that brilliance spread for us. The sun sinks lower until it reaches the windows of the office buildings across the river, and shatters into a mosaic of light. A cathedral, casting its light across the river in wavery patterns of radiance. I can't speak. A holy moment, because here we are, all together, safe at last.

"Dad, look!" I finally say. What I mean is, the world is still a beautiful place. You still have your life. I'm feeling expansive, blessed in some way. The office building is a cathedral now. I take this as a sign that everything will be all right. But of course he doesn't even know all the things he's lost, with losses still to come. I'm not the one sitting in the wheelchair trying to make sense of the menu. It's all too much. He blinks and says nothing. He's holding on to the armrests of his wheelchair, as if he can't quite trust the floor yet. He looks around, astonished. Life as it had been, before.

The server comes around to take our orders. He starts with my mother. She'll have the cod in sour cream and dill sauce, Caesar salad to start. She's been looking forward to this dinner as sort of a graduation, a commencement of good things to come. She starts to order a margarita, then changes her mind. Just water, thanks, she says. Better keep all her faculties intact, better not get a little fuzzy around the edges just yet. I wonder what she's been eating for dinner these past weeks. Hospital cafeteria food for days, sometimes a quick dinner with my uncle at Rosauer's, a half sandwich, cup of soup. I wonder if she's lost weight. "I'm going to really enjoy this dinner," she announces with formality.

Now the server looks at me. I don't care what I order. It's enough to just be here. So I pick the first thing my eyes light upon. I'll have the salmon, I say, but hold the vermouth butter, please, and extra vegetables, instead of the potatoes. Garden salad with blue cheese dressing on the side. Suddenly it occurs to me that I am only a kinder version of my difficult uncle.

My husband orders a steak, baked potato. Nothing held back, nothing on the side. He's a predictable, meat-and-potatoes kind of guy, but orders coffee instead of the Merlot, since he's the designated driver, and tonight everybody's on alert. He'd never order a steak if our daughter were here. He has always honored Courtney's vegetarian sensibility, though he grew up on a Colbert, Washington, farm. He'd helped his father milk the cows before school and after; birth the calves; castrate the males; butcher the steers; slaughter the pigs; feed the chickens; gather the eggs; mend the fences; build the barns; plow and spring-tooth harrow the fields; cut the hay and rake it into rows; separate the milk; churn it into butter. Nobody had to teach him the facts of life. But for his daughter's sake, he'd order down the food chain, though Courtney herself saw little hierarchy. If it had to die first, she would not eat it.

Then it's my father's turn. He's been staring at the menu as if he'd never seen one before. He turns the pages with his left hand. His right hand lies off duty against the tablecloth. Too many choices. They allow meal selection at the hospital, but it's always one thing or the other—beef stew or fried chicken, macaroni and cheese or pork chops. Now there's a frightening abundance of choices.

Of course he doesn't know what to order. Thus begins that sweet, sad effacement. "Grace, what do I want?" My mother looks startled, for a moment doesn't know what to say.

I wonder if this is the brain damage they sought and could not find—this inability to translate the words of the menu into desire. What do you want? What do you want? He wants to cut his own food, he wants to hold his fork in his right hand without trembling, he wants to sit in a regular chair, he wants to get up and take himself to the bathroom, he wants to be young and whole again. He wants his life with my mother to stretch out in front of him, days upon days of loving her as he used to.

"This is your night on the town, Homer," my mother says.

"Have the works, Dad. We're celebrating!" I say.

He picks up the menu again. It's shaking in his hands and he sets it down. "I don't know what I want." My father has always known what he wanted.

He looks at my mother blankly.

"You order for me."

She doesn't reveal a thing. I know how much she wants everything to be as it was, wheelchair notwithstanding. We are at a familiar and elegant and much-loved restaurant. He has crossed over to safety because here we are after all. Everything will be all right now, except for this problem with the menu. Give him a few moments. After all. He's been to the other side, and he's only just now making his way back. And there are so many choices. Pages and pages of choices—beef, poultry, lamb, pork, pasta, salads, appetizers, desserts, wines. I know how much she wants to rescue him, how much she wants him to prove to himself he needs no rescue anymore.

"Do you want a steak?" she says. But she's forgotten something else she never knew. If he orders a steak she will have to cut it.

"Okay," my father says. He closes the menu with his good hand and shuts his eyes.

My uncle is strangely silent. He looks at his brother leaning strangely to the right, sitting across the table in the wheelchair. I wonder what he's thinking. His worried look matches my father's. He orders the lamb. I want to stop him and say, "Uncle Henry! Remember last Christmas?"—that was before the stroke, which is how we measure time now—"when you ordered the lamb and it was rare and you shouted, 'I can't *eat* this, it's *raw*,'" and you sent it back and called the manager over and we all sat slumped in our chairs, waiting for your little fit to be over.

I wonder why he's ordered lamb. He doesn't even particularly like it. I'm the only symbolist at the table right now and can't help myself. Is that how he sees himself now, the sacrificial lamb on the altar of his brother's illness? Or how he has always seen himself in this world—the one twin sacrificed for the other, the one left out, left over, left behind? When you write this story, my mother says, figure out how Henry felt. She has given me some kind of permission here, to tell the story of my father and my uncle—or something I take as permission. But she is careful to add: "Don't put me in it."

I'm glad our daughter isn't here. She'd find a quiet way to prop the wine list in front of his plate, so she wouldn't see the raw lamb bleeding into the garlic mashed potatoes and broccoli, letting the pasta on her own plate grow cold. Vegetarians have it rough in the culinary world. How about a nice marinated tofu steak, thank you very much? No such chance. Her options were never more than fettuccine Alfredo, pasta primavera, or maybe a baked potato and salad, and no way to get any real protein.

Actually, I'm glad none of the children are here for this practice run. Dinners out with my uncle have always been fraught with disaster anyway. "I want *Roquefort* dressing, not blue cheese. Are you sure this is *Roquefort*? It tastes like *blue cheese*." Most of the time nobody knew what he was talking about, and when they say, "It's blue cheese, sir, that's all we have," he'd shake his head and say, "Well, all right then, if that's the best you can do." Then he'd order iced tea with *extra* lemon. "That means *three* pieces of lemon. I mean *three,* as in T-H-R-E-E." And all this on a good day. I fear I am making him sound like an ogre and wonder if I'll ever be able to explain how much we loved him. It was only the rough edges of old age. It was only his way of feeling important. He was only saying, "I'm here, I'm here! notice *me*."

When the lamb comes, and he can barely cut it, let alone chew it, he says nothing, but pushes it quietly to the side of his plate and sets down his knife and fork. He can't stop looking at his brother across the table, who is doing quite nicely on the bite-sized pieces of steak my mother has cut for him.

We're all beginning to relax. I look around and sigh. It feels almost normal. With a squint of the eye it almost does. We'll get there, I think, one of these days.

So that we won't have to get him in and out of the wheelchair to use the bathroom, something they do not want us to do yet, they fit him with something called an *external catheter*. I imagine it's like a sort of extended condom. Eventually, my mother will have to learn to put this on him when they want to go out, until he can manage the bathroom on his own. And it's one of the ways they will be intimate now. I have no idea and have never asked if their life as they had known it came to an end that Friday morning. It's outrageous to be wondering a thing like this when their lives have been altered so profoundly. Yet I tell myself it's a testimony to the extraordinary life my parents have led that I would wonder at all. Making love into their eighties. My mother made sure I knew how proud she was that he loved her like this.

It's dark now, and little white lights have come on all over the restaurant. Such enchantment for an October night. The restaurant lights flicker across the water. If I were my father I would never want to leave. But he does. He's had enough. He's had enough of everything. His back is tired and he's getting a little edgy. He's not followed the dinner conversation for quite a while now. But the bill is slow in coming, and my uncle is getting frantic. He feels everything my father feels. He begins to get up to find the manager to complain. My husband, who's sitting beside him, just turns and says, "No, Uncle Henry, you're not going to do that." My mother flashes him a thank-you look. We had wanted the evening to go on and on, and now we can't leave soon enough.

"Oh, I'm tired," my father says again. I think of the external catheter, then take my mind someplace else. If my father has the urge to use the bathroom he doesn't say. He's gone somewhere else, too. To the land of the invalid. *Invalid.*

Either way you say it, it means the same thing. Now he's listing to the right, and my husband gently repositions him. He wants his hospital bed, the pillows and covers just as he likes them, the TV bolted to the corner of the wall, the TV remote by his steady left hand, the nurses to pat him and take his temperature and blood pressure and listen to his heart and tell him that all is well.

After

When he finally masters the stairs, all twenty-one of them, the railing in one hand, the hand crutch in the other, my mother a step behind him holding on to his belt, he graduates from the hospital bed in the downstairs den to the big guest room at the top of the stairs. This room had once belonged to my grandmother Edna, whom my children had always called "Grape," since none of them could say "great-grandmother" when they were learning to talk. My mother's mother, the one I did not love, had lived with my parents for twenty years of their married life, my Uncle Henry for the last twenty. For five overlapping years, they all lived together, before my grandmother died. Grape had slept upstairs in the master bedroom, and two floors away, my uncle slept in his little room in the basement; and so the peace was kept.

My parents have both been in training for weeks for this move upstairs. A physical therapist has come to the house three days a week to help them practice getting up the stairs to bed at night, down the stairs for the morning. He slept badly downstairs in that hospital bed away from her, though they had intercoms between them. I had nightmares of my mother rushing down the stairs to a frantic, middle-of-the-night call, tripping on the way. "Grace! Grace!" he called a few times over those weeks, though he tried never to disturb her sleep if he could manage on his own.

Now he sleeps in the large, king-size bed in the big guest room, Grape's old room, where he'd been busy working on his new book. But his sleeping habits have become so odd while he was in rehab, they decide for the time being any-way, that my mother will continue to sleep across the hall in what has always been their bedroom, a whisper away. In the hospital he slept with the TV on mute, his radio that played classical music all night long tucked against his pillow. The blue flicker of the screen says someone is home, someone is watching over him while he sleeps. And it gives a certain quality of light against the night because he can-not abide the darkness. My mother sleeps lightly in the room across the hall, listening for a crash or thud or groan or maybe just the whispery comfort of Bach through the air. Now I lay me down to sleep. If I die before I wake.

My father was always great with titles. He titled his book *Even Presidents Die,* but his publisher had changed it to *The Presidents' Last Years,* which I always thought was kind of a shame. His current project, before the stroke, was *Between the Old and the New: A Study of the Jewish People between the Old Testament and the New.* He wasn't his preacher father's son for nothing. Now the detritus of those research days lies stacked about the room where he sleeps. That's where we all are now, on the road somewhere between the old and the new.

My mother has taken down the card table he'd been using as a desk and put his papers and notes in the corner. His books lie in piles against the wall. She didn't want to remove this reminder of his former life. It's their hope, of course, that he'll one day be able to pick up a pen and begin writing again. Neither of them wants to contemplate his life without work.

We buy him a computer to send e-mail, give him something new to think about, and act as rehab for his right hand. Maybe he can type what his right hand can't write. But he doesn't seem to be able to learn the sequence of it and tires quickly. My daughter writes out directions as simply as they can be given, in a large, printed hand. But he can't remember them, can't hit the right combination of keys, and too often plunges the computer into such hieroglyphs that we can't find the way out for days.

Maybe he could dictate into a tape recorder. Hire a secretary to take notes.

Anything to keep him from slipping into despair. Though often he would say, in astonishment, "You know, I'm supposed to be depressed, but I'm not." Yet he has given it up, the dream of the book, too easily and with only a little regret. "I wanted to write that book," he would say nostalgically, now and then, but never with much conviction. I don't think he remembered what it was he really wanted to say. He's already living in that place between the old and the new. He doesn't know the shape or outline of this in-between place, where he is neither sick nor well, one thing or the other, this life or the next.

My father has stopped reading. We never knew exactly whether there really is some electrical connection in his brain that has gone out or whether he's just too tired to follow the words across the page. We listen closely when he talks to see what we can find out. He often darts from one subject to another, and we wonder whether his mind is standing still or racing forward. Or whether it's operating at light speed now and caught up in an inner life that words can barely hold. But then this too is normal for him, because his thoughts have always jumped from one thing to another without segue, as if he could think on multiple, simultaneous levels. But now he mostly sits in his chair in front of the TV, the remote in his good hand, flipping from station to station, the only way he can go someplace on his own.

After his stroke the quality of his thinking changes in ways that both elude and surprise us. His response to everything now comes from an emotional center, which only seems to grow as his other faculties diminish. He has entered more fully the world of faith and belief to the exclusion of all else. His vision of the world is becoming more elemental, simpler. A comfort is wrapping itself around him. He worries both more and less. He sleeps a lot. He cannot remember his dreams. He can't think in complex terms, cannot abide ambiguity. He feels God closer now. "Let not your heart be troubled. Neither let it be afraid." It was what my preacher grandfather had said to my father sometimes to comfort him into sleep, and what my father had said to me.

Because my father's handwriting is not legible anymore, he persuades my mother, now and then, to write checks to an organization that sends Bibles to Russia, in exchange for a prayer cloth to be sent to him upon receipt of the check. I'm aghast at these things and don't understand their value as comfort to him, not that it matters in the least so long as my parents aren't using money they do not have. I am learning too slowly what things matter and what things do not. That he is not my intellectual father anymore shocks and saddens me. It's just another way we are losing him. I don't know that he is being honed, sharpened, purified as it were, down to his essence—that everything else is falling away. I have his genes. I have passed them on to my children. We will take good care of them for as long as we can until it is our turn to follow the circle of life to its inevitable conclusion.

There's no time I call now that my father doesn't answer the phone. It means he's in the family room, in the chair by the phone on the end table right next to where he's sitting. What else is there to do, anchored as he is to that maroon easy chair? Yet he's so proud to tell us how he can make seventeen circuits using just his hand crutch—from the family room through the kitchen, dining room, living room, and back to his chair. My mother has come to trust this circuit, and it's a testament of her faith in him, in progress, in faith itself, that she can now go up to her chair in the bedroom and read a little, away from the ever-present television set, which more often than not these days is tuned to a televangelist whom she cannot abide.

When the revivalist shouts, "Be *healed*. Stand up and walk for *Jesus*," my father pushes himself up out of his chair and takes a few steps unaided toward the television set. He is told by his doctors never to do this, by his physical therapist never to do this, but now and then he cannot resist those Southern cadences that reach something beyond reason or intelligence, back to his boyhood growing up in the Deep South as a preacher's son, in that little Free Methodist parsonage in St. Petersburg, Florida. That he is lulled to safety by those rhythms is all right by me.

So that is why it's a deep and heartless blow when the physical therapist releases my father from any further physical therapy. His insurance will not pay for any more sessions, which of course means that the therapist believes he will never be any better than he is right now. Everything that follows will be a turning backward. The miracle of the exercise bike, the stepping up and stepping down, the leg lifts, the arm curls, the right hand ball squeezes—all those lifts and stretches and tugs and pulls that will rewire the circuitry in his brain and place the desire in his heart against the betrayals of the body are past—they have done all they can reasonably do.

Something profound changes in my father after that. Not so many circuits with the hand crutch, no more walking toward the television with his arms stretched wide when the televangelist calls to him, "Be healed, my child, in the name of Jesus be healed." He knows somewhere deep inside that he is never going to be healed. The prayer cloth, just a humble square of muslin after all, lies in the end table drawer, to be pulled out once in a while in the night. What was there to place one's hope in now?

Months follow months as they struggle to stay in that three-story house so far away from us. "I'm keeping my head above water, but just barely," my mother confesses late one night. My uncle had given up driving several years ago, though his beige Chevy Caprice sits in the garage, his driver's license still tucked away in his wallet. He didn't say, "I'm never going to drive again." It was just that once coming home from a doctor's visit across town, he felt dizzy and suddenly couldn't remember where he was. Nobody had to wrench the keys away or threaten him with incompetence. It was just a sad, gentle erasure, possible only because my mother, always the best driver of the three of them, could still drive, but as we soon learned, not without peril.

Now it's February and Spokane is deep in the grip of winter. I've flown over from Seattle to spend the weekend, check on things, see if I can help out, as the mountain passes are still treacherous. I've told them not to bother coming out to the airport. Not knowing what those roads would be like, I'd take a cab. But they insist. Their daughter come to see them. Of course they would be there. They would not miss a moment of her. We would stop for dinner, celebrate.

I toss my bag in the trunk and slide into the backseat with my uncle, give everybody kisses and hugs. I notice the change right away. My mother is in the driver's seat, my father next to her. She's driving—that is, she's steering the car and using the gas and brake pedals. But my *father* is shifting the gears.

So this is how things have changed in the weeks between one visit and another. They take me out to dinner the next night and it is the same. My father picks up the garage door opener with his left hand and presses the switch. It's like the television remote. It's something he can make happen, something he can do. So the garage door scrolls up across the ceiling, a curtain rising onto the ordinary, perilous world.

"*Ready?*" my father says.

"Ready," my mother answers.

"Ready, Henry?" my father says to my uncle, who's riding shotgun in the backseat.

"Ready."

With the walker tucked away in the trunk, and my uncle's cane on the floor beside him, they're as ready as they can be. My mother hurt her shoulder several years before and cannot, without pain, shift the gears anymore, nor can she turn her head easily to look over her left shoulder. But my father can manage this with his left arm, and since the good left arm is closest to the gearshift anyway, he can manage this quite well—though it's easy to imagine him getting confused and putting the gear into drive instead of reverse and taking out the garage. But it's something he can do for her, when there is so little left he can do.

And so with his "good" arm, my father shifts into reverse as my mother steps on the gas pedal and away we go. My uncle turns to the left. "Okay my way," he says.

My father is looking to the right. "Okay my way," he echoes.

My mother is concentrating on the rearview mirror, though my uncle is also supposed to help her look behind. By now they are well practiced at this, and that calms me a little. Yet my heart is racing, and I can only think oh my, oh my. So this is what we've come to. We get halfway downtown before I realize I've forgotten to put on my seatbelt.

It is a choreography of safety and love, though they would never have recognized it at the time. Together the three of them can get backed out of the garage, down the driveway, and out into the street. Together, the three of them can make it across town down wintry streets, to the places of their communal life that month by month become increasingly circumscribed.

I wish them all the traveling mercies in the universe as they make their way down those icy streets to and from the church and grocery store and pharmacy and a few favorite restaurants with handicapped access, and a thousand doctor's appointments. Taken together, they are complete. They have everything they need—arms, legs, eyes. It's such an emblem of their strange and valiant life, yet I wonder how they will survive the losses to come, how any of them will do without the others.

There are stairs everywhere, nothing to think about when they bought the house twenty years ago, long after I'd moved out to go to college and get married. They could do those stairs two at a time. In fact, those stairs, separating the three floors of the house, were one of the reasons they bought it to begin with.

My parents and I had moved to Washington State because my father had been offered a history professorship at Whitworth College in Spokane, but also because my mother's parents had moved to Walla Walla from Pennsylvania a few years before. Spokane was a only a four-hour trip to Walla Walla, not six days by car, if they should need us. My grandfather's dynamite-moving business was no job for a man with a bad heart, so when offered a job with a realty firm in Walla Walla, my grandparents moved West, and in 1955 we followed. By 1957 they were living with us, and by 1958 my grandfather was dead.

And then in 1977, when my uncle moved to Spokane from Michigan after his retirement, my parents sold the house they and my grandmother and I had lived in during my growing-up years, and moved into a new three-story house, which would accommodate them all.

Because he was my father's twin and because he had nowhere else to go, my parents made a little apartment for my uncle downstairs, with a bedroom and private bath. But it was twenty stairs down and twenty stairs up, and now he has his own problems with navigation. Yet those stairs kept things as easy among them as was possible, given the difficult personalities of my grandmother and my uncle.

Grape commanded the family room in the mornings, and had her own chair, where she watched quiz shows on TV. My mother said it was one of the things that kept her so sharp. She would shout out the answer before the contestant did, and clap her hands when she was right, which was a lot of the time. Her soap operas she watched upstairs in her bedroom. My mother had said, "If God ever wants to punish me, he'll send my mother to live with me." She didn't really believe this, but it gave her the comic distance to get through the days and weeks and years as she tried to love her mother and couldn't, though she watched over her with exquisite care.

Grape gouged countertops and cabinets with her slapdash ways in the kitchen, which they had pretty much turned over to her, so she would have an arena of her own. So she made the family dinner every night, which was nice for her and a blessing for my parents, coming home after a long day at work.

My mother had long suspected that Grape steamed open their mail when they were at work. My mother once plotted with my uncle when he lived in Michigan to send them a letter saying he'd run off to Las Vegas and gotten married to a showgirl, to see if Grape would trap herself. That idea was great fun among my parents and my uncle, but the letter never did get written, as far as I know.

To get to the garage, my uncle would have to walk through the family room, where my grandmother watched her quiz shows. I'd seen him steel himself against the coming cross-examination, one of the battles for control they fought in mostly little ways.

"Where are you going?" she'd bark as he headed for the door.

"*Out.*"

"Well then when will you be back?"

"I don't know."

"Well you must have some idea."

"I have no idea *whatsoever.*" And he'd slam the door.

But during those five or so years when both my uncle and my grandmother lived with my parents, my uncle took my grandmother to her church across town every Sunday and picked her up after it was over. It was one way he could help out my parents. I can see him driving stony faced, while she kept up her usual rush of talk. My parents used to wonder how he kept from driving off the road. But he did this willingly and without complaint. After she died in 1982, he said to my parents, "You know, she never thanked me once." But he called her a respectful "Mrs. Piper." Not "Edna," and never "Mom," which was my father's custom.

My father tried his best to protect me from Grape's meddling ways, and truly, I remember little of her interference when we all lived together during my teenage years. And then I got married and soon was coming home to visit from Seattle with our babies. How she loved them when they were so little and could love her back unconditionally. I was happy I could give her something at last, when I had felt such guilt all those years for never loving her in my secret heart.

Out of all the sixty-six years of their marriage, my parents had shared their lives with others for over forty of them. It's a complicated thing to explain, except to say that my parents felt they could do no other. So it was stairs all around, and it was stairs that allowed them to live together in the same house for all those years. Now those stairs were every bad dream, with no end to the ways any one of them could fall.

Each morning of that weekend home, I watch my father coming down those long stairs in the morning, all dressed and ready to go, my mother in her pajamas and robe. She's dressed him first, as he won't make his way back up those stairs for anything but to go to bed. And there he goes, step by treacherous step, his crutch in one hand, the other hand holding fast to the railing. My mother follows behind him, holding on to his belt. If he were to begin to topple forward on the trip down, her instructions are to pull back hard on his belt, and sit right down. I do not picture this all those nights trying to fall asleep, three hundred miles away on the other side of the mountains. I only see them toppling one over the other, coming to rest in a fatal, tangled heap at the bottom of the stairs. I close my eyes against this every morning and say a prayer for their safe passage through the day, safe passage up the stairs at night.

Then as I'm getting ready for bed the last night of my weekend visit, still haunted by this new thing—this imperiled way of driving—I wonder if there are other changes I've yet to notice. I'm convinced beyond all doubt that they need to be in a safe place where there is no need of driving anywhere, no need for stairs. Which of course has been the subject of endless discussion even before the stroke, but so far to no avail.

My parents had even put deposit money down on a retirement community in Issaquah, just outside Seattle, then backed out at the last minute. Ed and I had driven out and measured the rooms and drawn up floor plans. I think the four of us looked at five places before my father's stroke. Then my father passed the torch on to me. My parents and uncle didn't have the money to buy in, which was the only way they could go to a retirement community with a nursing home attached. It was all a crazy business, and my mother just said, "Don't worry about the nursing home part. Just find a place with Assisted Living." That's as far as she could get her thinking to go. "We'll figure it out if the time comes." That was fine by me. I couldn't abide the vision of any of them in such a place either. Even after the stroke, I told myself I would never permit it.

During my visits home to Spokane, including this one, I stay upstairs in the little guest room with the twin beds and the closet. I go into the bathroom of the big bedroom, now my father's bedroom, and notice a chalky glass sitting on the counter by the sink. I take it downstairs and put it in the dishwasher. I'm trying to find little, unobtrusive ways to help out. For a flicker of a second I wonder what has happened to my mother's tidy ways, but considering everything, it's a wonder things are as tidy as they are. A little while later my mother comes to the head of the stairs and calls down after me. "Did you take the Maalox glass?" My mother's voice is shaky with anger.

"Yeah," I say, "I put it in the dishwasher."

I can see even from the bottom of the stairs that she is near tears. "There's no glass for his Maalox now," she says. I have never seen her this way.

"Oh I'm sorry," I say, "I thought it needed to be washed. I'll bring another one right up."

"But that's the Maalox glass."

"Can't he have his Maalox in another glass?"

"It's the only one that's the right size."

"Okay," I say, thinking of the rows and rows of glasses in the cupboard. "I'll wash it out and bring it up." I do not recognize her. This tightening is another thing that has happened these past weeks in my absence.

33

Then it's an hour or so later and my mother is getting ready to help my father to bed. I watch her leaning over to adjust the bedding in that king-size bed my husband and I used to sleep in when we visited, before my father needed a large bed of his own. She's leaning over, adjusting the bedding, and I notice how she winces when she stands up.

"Hey, Ma, let me do that."

"You wouldn't know how," she says coolly.

How hard can this be? I almost say, but do not. But she sees my look and feels she must explain the complexities of my father's bed making—how the covers have to be loosely tucked, except for the foot of the bed on the side where my father sleeps, where they have to be completely untucked. He doesn't like the feeling of being trapped by anything, even the bedclothes, and considering all the ways he's trapped already, it's a small thing that's become a big thing, which characterizes so much of his life now.

Finally she sits down on the edge of the bed and I sit down beside her. We can hear the television from downstairs, where my father sits, waiting to be brought up to bed. She reaches back, smoothes out the covers. "Even then, when people didn't know so much or talk about it," she says without segue, "we never made love but that your father didn't please me." She smiles at me, and for a moment we just sit there saying nothing. "I'm glad I can tell you this."

"Me too," I say.

"You know he was always faithful to me."

I can only nod because my eyes are spilling over with tears and I turn away.

She has not said this part of their life together is over, but her use of the past tense sounds like it, and I can't think of a way to ask. Later, just before she goes to bed, she pops her head into the room where I'm already in bed, reading a magazine. It's near midnight. "Well, we'll just have to stay here till we *croak*. Then you can figure out what to do with all this." I know what she means. All three floors.

The garage. The yard. So much for that argument for moving into a retirement community my father and I had been pitching for years now.

I laugh. "Ma," I say. It's not really a laugh. She loves to use the word *croak* for death. *Kick the bucket* is my father's expression. Anything but *dying, died, dead.* If you knew my cool, sophisticated mother, and her competence in all things, you would know what the unraveling of her composure by that Maalox glass was all about. I knew then that they were teetering on the edge, and my job was to get them out of there as soon as I could.

It wasn't that she didn't want to move. She just couldn't figure out how to get from one place to the other. She'd had a kind of stroke too. She'd lost a certain flexibility of thought and emotion. She was living from hour to hour, a stairs' tumble away from the end. In her former life, my mother had been dean of women at Greenville College in Greenville, Illinois. She had a master's in guidance and counseling from Washington University in St. Louis. When we moved to Spokane, she supervised all the counselors and psychologists for the Spokane School District. She'd been president of the Spokane Education Association. She was named administrator of the year for the state of Washington and received her award from the governor. I loved to think of her in this way, all the things she'd done so competently and without ego. Now here we were. Please don't be old, Ma. Don't do it. No reason to go and do that.

My uncle had lived with my parents all those years before my father's stroke, but now I can see how they have become a threesome in ways they never were before. At night, my uncle carries my mother's special back pillow for her up the stairs to her bedroom. A little gesture that is gallant, quiet, respectful. I have often wondered if he had ever fallen in love with her too. If he had, he kept his own counsel. I always imagined that he loved her immensely, but as one would a beloved sister. My uncle's heart was outside my knowing in this and many other things.

My uncle was held firmly in the center of their lives, yet I think he always felt a certain tenuousness in his position. They were a couple and he was the one they added on. He tried very hard to be worthy of inclusion, though more often than not he was a trial for both my parents. How could he not be? It was unusual, and perhaps people talked, my mother living with two identical men.

Even into their eighties, my father and my uncle were virtually identical. The same broad face, the same wavy dark hair, though now mostly gray, the same broad smile, the slightly aquiline, classic nose, the same wide laugh. And the same passionate love of American history, my father as a college professor and my uncle as a high school teacher, then administrator.

Back home in Michigan, my uncle was a man about town. Lots of girlfriends. Best friends with the mayor. History teacher, of course, but also championship debate coach, director of Special Ed kids, administrator, teacher of the year so many times they finally retired the award.

Such a big fish in little, aristocratic Marshall, Michigan, where he lived in a rented, upstairs bachelor apartment in the home of Mary and Helen Edgerton, two elderly and wealthy maiden ladies, until they died. He was their almost son and they were his virtual aunts if not his mothers. They were going to will the house to him if he would stay in Michigan to keep it, but after they died he did not want to stay, and so when he retired, he moved to Spokane to live with my parents.

But here in Washington, he was mainly the twin of Homer Cunningham, whom people were always mistaking him for. So he grew a moustache. Besides, he didn't want any crazy people mistaking Henry for Homer. There was a reason why my father kept that shotgun of my grandfather's in the upstairs closet.

My father was chair of both the History and American Studies Departments at Whitworth College in those days, but he counseled students as well. So there he was when Eddie Gray, another outcast of the universe, made his way to my father's office door. He said his wife had left him to move back with her parents and kid brother and sister. "She won't do what I tell her," he told my father. "So sometimes when she's washing her hair, I hold her head under the water." What my father heard that day chilled him so much he made arrangements for Eddie Gray to see a psychiatrist the next day, an appointment that was never kept. Then he called Eddie Gray's wife and told her to get a restraining order *now*, and get a dog. A big dog.

So one fall evening in 1958 when my father was watching television and a news bulletin came across the screen about a north-end Spokane mass murder, my father rushed to the phone and called Eddie Gray's wife to be sure they were all safe, that it wasn't what in his gut he knew it was, and a detective answered the phone and told him that the wife was dead, the mother and father were dead, but the two kids were safe. They'd hidden themselves under a bed and were spared.

"Don't worry," the detective said, "this type always goes off somewhere and kills himself." My father said, "No, he won't. He'll go off somewhere, but he won't kill himself. You'll have to do it for him."

And so my father waited up all night with my grandfather's rifle across his lap well into the morning when they finally caught Eddie Gray just as my father had said, holed up in the woods, armed with a gun. I don't have a vivid memory of the night with my father keeping watch with my grandfather's shotgun, no vivid memory of the dark thing that might be just outside the window, did not imagine a heavy boot kicking in the front door and firing away. I just remember the fear in my father's eyes, and his clean white dress shirt as I hugged him goodnight.

My mother went to the trial the day my father gave his testimony. She watched Eddie Gray's sloping shoulders as he sat there hunched over, sobbing into a white handkerchief. His flat, gray, red-rimmed eyes, his Brylcreem hair. After the trial Eddie Gray said that if Homer Cunningham hadn't interfered, he wouldn't have had to kill them, though my father was the principal witness for the defense, and was the one who saved his life. My father, who would have shot him dead to save us, believed that even Eddie Gray was worthy of redemption.

Twenty-five years later, in her last day in office, the governor of our state commuted the life sentence of Eddie Gray. He had been rehabilitated, according to the governor's office. But what was broken in Eddie Gray could not be fixed. And so a few weeks later, sometime in the late 1980s, when my father got a phone call, saying his daughter in Seattle (that would be me) had been kidnapped, his mind went first to Eddie Gray, who had always blamed my father for the miseries of his life, who had never wavered from the view that if it hadn't been for my father's interference, he wouldn't have had to do the terrible thing he did.

"We've got her," the reedy voice said. "You'll never see her again."

"Oh, how it felt to have lost you," he told me later. "Never to see your face again on this earth, I could not bear it." But I had not been kidnapped. I was found safe after all, sitting in the back of my classroom, listening to a student panel discuss Toni Morrison's *Beloved*, which explains my secretary's panic at not seeing me at first glance. But as days passed safely one after the other, Eddie Gray faded from view and finally disappeared from our lives altogether. But in the closet of that little room where I stay when I visit, there is my grandfather's rifle, propped back in the corner behind my father's suits. That gun both comforts and haunts me, though I try not to remember it's there.

Now there was no need of a moustache to tell my uncle and my father apart. My father was the one with the hand crutch, the walker, the wheelchair. And now here we were again, facing down that most ancient of enemies, coming around some corner any day now on a whisper or the wind.

From the beginning of their life together, my uncle tried to fit into my parents' lives. He had his little chores, which he did happily. And after my father's stroke, he was indispensable. He set his alarm to get up in the morning before everyone else, and lay three small juice glasses in a row on the counter, lined up three spoons, three dishes, got out the oatmeal, the butter, the juice, while my mother got my father all dressed and ready for the day. Then my mother would come down, holding on to my father's belt, as they made their way step by step downstairs. My father sat in his TV chair watching the news while my mother made the oatmeal—with hot water and butter instead of milk. The same with Shredded Wheat. I couldn't imagine it. No milk, no brown sugar. She preferred the sweeter version, also, but it was too much trouble to do things separately, just for herself. "Oh, it's just another one of their *Southern things*," my mother would wryly say, along with white rice, okra, grits, and fried chicken, all of which she willingly cooked for them, though she hated rice and grits and okra. It was just another way she effaced herself all those years.

The twins were born in Athens, Georgia, just outside Atlanta, but they spent their boyhood in St. Petersburg, Florida, where their preacher father had been assigned a new church. They were the boys of summer, racing through the sunlight across the hot sand in their rush to that wide ocean. They were the boys of summer year after year until their father's reassignment to the seminary in Spring Arbor, Michigan, when the boys were teenagers. How they must have missed the ocean and the palm trees and the avocados and oranges hung low from their backyard trees. They must have been doted on by their father's Free Methodist church congregation—they were *identical twins*, after all—but as Preacher's Kids, or PKs, they had to conform to exemplary standards. Yet some of their antics were so clever they must have drawn a smile from their father, if not their solemn mother.

Homer and Henry hated Harold Mathewson, a member of their father's congregation, known for his piety, his long prayers, and his Sunday afternoon strolls in his straw hat and white suit. He was always clearing his throat and looking down his nose at the boys, as if he could read their scheming minds. "Are you boys in the hands of the Lord? Or are you in mortal danger of damnation?"

"No, sir," they said in unison, tucking in the smile. They loved the ambiguity, the way it turned both ways.

"Well, you boys be good now," he said, pointing at each boy's chest with his walking stick.

It didn't take them long to plot their revenge. They took some fishing wire and stretched it across the sidewalk from one tree to another just above his head, right in the path of his Sunday afternoon walk, and a few yards farther on, they did the same with another pair of trees. Then they waited in the bushes until he rounded the corner, tapping his walking stick as he went, all puffed up in his Sunday best. Suddenly his hat flew off. He jerked his head up, looked around, batted at the air. Now who had knocked off his hat? He picked it up and settled it just so, straightened his tie, and went on his way. A few yards on, that hat flew off again. Then arms, hands, walking stick all raging at the empty air, and now actual *swear* words only the boys could hear as they hid in the bushes, doubled over. Double trouble. Double joy. One happy, one sad. One bright, one dark. On days like that, they were two halves of a greater whole.

In their growing-up years, no one but their parents could tell them apart, and so they were always switching themselves around. They must have loved and hated that they were so interchangeable. At Greenville College, where they spent their undergraduate years, they would go to classes for each other, and in a pinch, take each other's tests. They conspired to tell their father that their fines for overdue books were really not fines at all, but "Library Laboratory Fees." They were men about campus at that small Free Methodist college, just east of St. Louis, where my parents met, where I was born, where my father began his teaching career, and where I spent my very early years.

My Pennsylvania-born mother often explained my father's ways to me like this: "He was born just outside *Atlanta*, Ann. He grew up in the *South*. That's why he's so protective." For a long time I didn't understand what one had to do with the other, until a memory rose up from my childhood. Each Christmas when we lived in Illinois, my parents and my uncle and I would make our way to Florida to visit my uncle's namesake, Uncle Henry, Aunt Susie, and their daughter, grown-up Cousin Dorothy, to sit in their backyard in the sun and talk of old times. I turned cartwheels and somersaults while they talked, waiting for it to be time to go swim in the ocean. The South was as strange and distant from my Midwestern existence as I could imagine—an exotic place with alligators and crocodiles and flamingos and creepers and vines. In the South *dinner* was at noon, and *supper* in the evening. Words melted into each other with soft caramel beginnings and endings, sweet honeysuckle shimmered in the air, avocado and tangerine trees gathered themselves into half-moons of shade and under them we had our iced tea and biscuits. My Great Uncle Henry was a carpenter by trade and had built his house to withstand any storm blowing in from the Gulf. It was hurricane proof, he always said, a house safe from everything but death.

We were sitting on a wide, white porch when Great Aunt Susie picked me up and held me tight, *Oh my child, my child,* she said, before I could respectfully wriggle away. As the story goes, Aunt Susie held three-year-old Dorothy just like this after her two babies died. Dorothy was her third baby and the only living child. "Dorothy is the oldest child I ever had," she said. "I'm not going to ever let her go." And she never did. Dorothy, or Dot, as we called her, never left that house built for hurricanes, and lived there into her old age.

By the fierce way Aunt Susie held me, I knew what Dorothy must have felt like all those years. When I was three I almost died of pneumonia. My father held me just like Aunt Susie had held Dorothy and said, *My child, my child.* He would have loved it if I'd never left home. When I was growing up my father caught me in a net of love and fear. "Now don't just go off on your own. Stay with the group," my father was always saying. When I was all grown up and a Hemingway scholar going off to Cuba for the first time, he told me the same thing. "You know how you like to just go off. Stay with people you know." Cuba was a far country. I would be so far outside his protection he wouldn't even know what to warn me of. But I had learned my lesson well. I knew how to be afraid of many things. Yet in 1995 I did go to Cuba, even if it was with a group—the first group of Hemingway scholars to be guests of the Cuban government at that. Now this journey toward death my father and I were taking was a far country, all right. There was no group to shelter me now.

My father's Southern ways shadowed my growing up in small matters only, because I grew into my selfhood beneath the canopy of his abiding love. But at the time I often felt his protectiveness wrenchingly. By then my father had taken a position in the History Department at Whitworth College in Spokane, where I spent my grade school and teenage years. The blight of those years was my father's rule against school dances. When I was crowned Spokane "Lilac Princess," something my children have always found outrageously funny, my father gave me a dozen red roses and a card that said, "For my Beautiful Princess." So I was my father's Princess, just like daddies' little girls are supposed to be. But I preferred to be his Pill, not his Princess.

Yet his pride in me was shadowed by his fear that there would be a Lilac Festival formal dance I would be required to attend. Something happened when boys and girls danced together that he could only allude to darkly. His rule forbidding me to attend high school dances came from long, anguished nights he spent balancing my adolescent happiness against the dangers he saw waiting for me in those dimly lit gyms. My uncle agreed. In fact, it may have been his idea to begin with. After all, he supervised high school dances all the time. Terrible things happen at those dances. So the twins decided they would protect me from myself and all those boys who would line up to dance with me and do unspeakable things to me in the dark corners of the gym or in the backseat of a car in the school parking lot. In the South men protected their women from other men and, in a certain sense, from themselves, too.

But after much pleading and many tears on my part, my father allowed me to go to one dance—my Junior Prom, if I promised never to ask him again. I could have the dress (tastefully modest), the corsage, the cookies and punch. I could ride in the car with the boy. I could sit next to him. I could have my picture taken with him. But I could not actually *dance* with him. My mother told me she had been forbidden to go to school dances by her father too. Her father took her hunting in the hills of Pennsylvania, and taught her to change a tire. If she was going to drive, she had to be able to change a tire. He was preparing her for life in the world as an independent woman. When she became a social worker traveling those wintry back roads in Pennsylvania, before she married my father, she could change a tire if she had to, thanks to my grandfather. He was quiet and gentle and loving, but in this matter of dances, he was like my father. He was protecting her from things outside her girlhood knowledge.

But my mother, rebel that she was, snuck out and went to dances anyway, and learned all the latest steps. She would not be left out. Her secret desire all her life was to learn to tap dance, but no sneaking out would be able to teach her that. I was no such rebel. I did not sneak out to dances or to anything else. I toed the line because I knew how much it hurt my father to say no to me. So I sat in a folding chair with my date beside me, until the music pulled him away from me and out onto the dance floor with the other girls.

My only visit to Atlanta was with my parents a couple of years before my father's stroke. I was an English professor by then, at the University of Puget Sound, and in Atlanta to give a conference paper at the South Atlantic Modern Language Association. I had fallen in love with Hemingway my sophomore year in college, and wondered where my affection would take me, or whether it was only a schoolgirl crush. But late in my graduate school career it was still Hemingway and no other. So I'd written my doctoral dissertation on the development of his short stories, and now here I was.

And after my talk, we all were going to visit the "Atlanta cousins," none of whom I had ever met. We were going to stay in my conference hotel, then move to my cousin Omie's house just outside Atlanta. My topic was "Hemingway and Androgyny," a topic I had spent most of the summer wrestling with. This was still relatively new and inflammatory terrain, and I was worried how it would go over with the "old boys" in the Hemingway Society, who would surely rise up to defend Papa against the outrageous claims that Hemingway also had a deeply feminine side. And though I worried about this, I also worried that if that old guard attacked me, my father would stand up and shout, "Stop picking on *my girl!*" He was proud of my academic life, proud that I had gone into college teaching as he had, and relieved I had not gone into show business, as I had wanted to do from the first time he took me to a circus. I couldn't tell him now that I was afraid he might embarrass me. So I asked my parents not to come to my presentation because it would make me too nervous, and they gently said it was all right, and never showed their disappointment. So the afternoon of my paper they checked out of the hotel and went on to my cousin's house while I stayed at the hotel waiting to give my late-afternoon talk.

My father had never understood my love of literature. "Why don't you go into *history* instead?" he was always teasing me. Even though he did not see the connection between us, I did. After all, my specialty was *American* literature. I had even done my master's thesis on Jonathan Edwards, the same figure my father had devoted part of his doctoral dissertation to, though in a vastly different way. He did not understand literature in the way I read it or taught it or wrote about it, and he was chastened by the fact that these things I loved remained outside his understanding.

My presentation was applauded that late afternoon in Atlanta, Georgia. I was elected chair of next year's session. I had an expensive dinner by myself at the hotel, while my parents had dinner with the Atlanta relatives. I brought along a good book for company and told myself what a fine time I was having. Then I went back up to my hotel room, saw the other bed where they had been, and knew what a terrible mistake I had made. How my father would have loved seeing me a great success. There would never be another chance. It wouldn't have mattered to me or to him if he hadn't understood the subtleties of androgyny in Hemingway.

I was always a little sad our family was so small, and at times I was lonely. The Atlanta cousins would make me a part of a big family too. There was my father's cousin Joe and his five kids; his favorite cousin, Omie, and her husband, Elmer; and their son, Ed, the multimillionaire, who'd made his fortune "in garbage" as his mother laughingly put it. But the money came from mysterious dealings his parents either were not privy to or did not understand. Exporting and importing, things going out and things coming in. Tony Soprano comes to mind, and all the money to be made in "waste management." My cousin of the Atlanta mafia.

The next day, Omie drove us to the Atlanta Cyclorama, which depicted the Battle of Atlanta. The only history I knew of the city I'd gotten from *Gone With the Wind*. We settled ourselves into tiered seats on a revolving platform in the center of an enormous room that held a mural over forty feet high and almost three hundred and sixty feet around. The lights dimmed and the Battle of Atlanta passed before us. I remember sitting by my father, watching the Civil War float by and my father pointing out the plaster of paris model of Clark Gable. I remember Clark Gable but nothing else about the mural. I remember thinking: This is where my father was born. This is where he came from. These Atlanta cousins are people I belong to because they belong to him. So the South was inside my father and my uncle, and inside me. But I would never be here with him like this again.

Now how strange to watch them eating breakfast all together like that, my uncle and mother in their pajamas and robes, my father all dressed up as though he had a big day ahead. Everything they did now was like this. In this slow-motion dance of their lives there was a certain beauty, if only you could forget the fragility of it, the attenuation.

I see Uncle Henry so clearly now, in the morning, with his slept-on hair sticking every which way, his worn-down-at-the-heels brown leather slippers, his baggy pajamas gathered up and pinned at the waist with a big safety pin, his brown cotton robe—setting out things for breakfast. In the bottom of his closet are several pairs of new pajamas in their Christmas boxes, a new pair of slippers, a new robe. Why this reluctance to give up the familiar, this determination to hold on to it no matter what? Maybe the feel and smell of these old clothes reassured him that things would not change while he slept, when enormous changes seemed to threaten at every turn. An incantation for safe passage through the night.

My uncle cleaned the kitchen three times a day, took out the trash, got the mail, helped my mother bring in the groceries. He tried to be useful, unobtrusive in their lives, aware that he was a guest even so, and living there out of their love for him.

And all the things he did by night my parents knew nothing of. We had seen him travel through the house in the dark, checking for any flaw in its defenses, double-checking the locks, the drapes, walking through room by room just to be sure. The old lamplighter himself, announcing to all sleepless souls, "Twelve o'clock and all is well, you can go to sleep now." He was their sentinel, their guardian, though they hardly knew it. Late one night over Christmas one year, the kids took kitchen things—a colander, Jell-O mold, rolling pin, an omelet pan—and put them in the sink, where he would find them in the morning when he got up to set out the things for breakfast, and wonder what had happened during the night. "What were you kids *doing* last night?" he said, shaking his head. "Cooking," they said. Now how had he missed it? He was the night watchman and all this had slipped by him. No wonder he went back to bed and slept till noon.

He kept a nickel-plated revolver in the top drawer of his dresser, which we did not find until we went through his things after he died. It was unloaded, and we never found any bullets. I don't think my uncle had ever fired at anything. With his lifelong vertigo, he would have probably only shot himself. But the poignancy of his safekeeping duties was not always apparent to my parents. He locked things up early and closed the drapes against the night far earlier than my mother wanted. She liked looking out at the streetlights, the people going by taking their dogs for walks. She wanted to delay that closed-in feeling for as long as possible.

For my mother, life had folded in upon itself and become a series of ever-repeating hours to get safely through. When you're treading water and getting no nearer the shore, there is no past, and the future cannot be imagined. But for my father, time was rushing forward and he could do nothing to stop it. He was imagining his death now, and I think preparing for it in little ways, both consciously and unconsciously. After so many things had gone wrong over the years, announcing themselves with alarm and then fading into a sort of chronic hum, like the static on his late-night TV—now this stroke might take him and leave my uncle with my mother.

The Ice Storm

In eastern Washington the winters are unforgiving and permit no missteps. All those times out to the car over the snowy, icy driveway, and all the walkways and stairways into and out of places that should have been shoveled and sanded but were not, my father with his walker, my uncle with his cane, my mother not so steady herself—and no one fell. They went on with their lives, to church, to restaurants, to doctors' appointments, to the pharmacy. And my mother, bundled up against the cold, to Albertson's for the weekly grocery shopping, which she had always done with my father, making her perilous way alone over the icy parking lot. And no one fell.

It's the middle of November in the second year of the stroke. The temperature, just at the edge of freezing, has turned the slanting rain to ice during the night, and an ice storm has swept across Spokane, toppling trees and cutting power to thousands of people, including my parents.

My father watches an ice-glazed pine tree fall in slow motion toward the house, taking out part of the deck in the process, landing a foot or two from the room where he sits, looking out in astonishment. Trees fall all over the city just like that, breaking circuits, connections, and putting out the lights. No heat, no lights, no hot water, no hot food. Three people in their eighties wrapped up against a cold and wintry darkness as treacherous inside as it is outside. There must have been many such people stranded like this with no place to go.

"Can't you just go to a hotel?" I ask over the phone, barely holding my panic in check. But no, all the hotels are full, and there is no room in any inn anywhere.

So they sleep covered up in sweaters and coats and blankets all together in the family room. A neighbor brings them hot chili out of a thermos, and eventually, after the third night, invites them for a sleepover in their living room, which has a catalytic heater. The blackout stretches to five days, and more. Finally my mother finds a hotel with power, though at first they say they have no rooms. "My husband has had a stroke, we are in our eighties, we have nowhere else to go." And finally a room is found for them. Heat, lights, hot food, hot water, warm beds, television, radio. So my mother packs up all their supplies—a change of clothes, pajamas, medicines, the ubiquitous Depends discreetly tucked away in a cloth bag, the walker—the accoutrements of the life of the handicapped—and they make their treacherous way over icy streets across town.

Then my mother and my uncle get my father out of the car and onto his walker, which he inches toward the waiting hotel door and safety at last. The three of them stand there just inside the doors that close behind them and look into a lobby lit by candlelight. There is one lone employee at the desk. My mother marches across the lobby and stands there until he looks up. She is so angry and afraid she can hardly speak.

"But I *asked* you. I asked you if you had power and you said you did."

My mother can't remember what he said in response. But then there was really nothing to say. A mistake had been made. Someone had misspoken. We are so sorry.

Then they return as they had come, across the frozen city to their darkened, waiting house, no place to come home to now. I want to fly across the state and bring them over to Seattle. You read all the time of old people shut away in their apartments in the winter when the power goes out just slipping away in their sleep. But they say no, it would be too much trouble to get all packed up. The power has been out so long it's bound to come back any minute. It can't go on much longer.

It can go on forever. They were living in this dark and frozen place far from me. I could lose them. Every one of them. But they were valiant in their hope that even now, they—*the power crew? city officials? the National Guard? God Almighty?*—were reconnecting the circuitry that would rewire the city and cast out the dark.

I think of my father and wonder if the doctors would one day be able to reconnect the things that had been broken off by some ice storm in his brain that threw him into the dark. The comparison would not have occurred to me then. But here as before, I long for metaphor not science to describe what has happened to him. To see correspondences between the natural world and our lives is to see a pattern, even if that pattern is mortality. Two weeks later at Thanksgiving, Ed and I drive by fields of trees flattened by the ice, forests laid bare as in some scorching war. But as in a forest fire, the trees would eventually nourish the soil beneath them and give way to new life. The circuitry of the city will eventually be fixed, though in some areas not for weeks. But no restoration for my father. For him the trees are down for good.

So they huddle together in their family room and wait through that nuclear winter in front of an unlit fireplace, no one to get the wood, build a fire, keep it going. We would have to get them out of there one way or another, because now I know they can't survive another winter where they are. The precariousness of their footsteps through the winter ice and snow is beginning to convince even my mother how unsafe they are. At Thanksgiving, Ed and I buy a gas insert fireplace for that room where they stayed together those long dark days. It will give them some radiant heat and light even without power. That was something, at least—the illusion of coziness, of safety, of abiding life.

• • •

Then I find University House—the most beautiful retirement community I'd ever seen—and put their name on the waiting list. My mother actually mails in a deposit, a not inconsiderable sum. But it's the third time they've done all this, and nothing is for sure. And so we wait. I wonder how long they can wait before they'll be refused at the door. You have to know the name of the president, your social security number, and other things of little consequence. They wouldn't ask you to remember the name of your first love or heartbreak, or the names of your grandchildren, or your wife's favorite color.

"Annie, get us someplace safe," my father whispers over the phone every chance he gets. "We can't stay here much longer."

"I know," I say, "you're on that waiting list, remember?"

My uncle, of course, doesn't want to change a thing. He always says, "I think we're doing just fine right where we are." My mother is frozen into place. A three-story house with a lifetime's accumulation of things, a two-car garage, a big yard. She's hoping their name never comes up, that they will remain safely hidden somewhere in the middle of that waiting list, forever a possibility and no urgent reality. My mother believes she can keep things going where they are for as long as she needs to. Me, I count the days and weeks, pray for spring. I call the director of University House at least once a week about their status on the list, terrified they will be unable to cross over to safety in time.

For Christmas I persuade them to fly to Seattle, so they can see this place, only half an hour from our home, for themselves. My husband will fly over and pick them up, fly back with them, and then get them home the same way. I've taken pictures, drawn floor plans of the place I had found for them, more beautiful than I could ever have imagined a place such as this could be. It's a place worthy of them, full of life, beauty, art, and an intellectual community of people who have led interesting and powerful lives. It's a retirement community, not an *old folks' home*, and certainly not a nursing home. This seemed a plus to me at the time, short-sighted as we all were. I imagined the three of them living years in comfort and style, since there was no nursing home wing anywhere in sight.

My father's wearing his camel blazer with the suede trim, his brown wool pants, his brown oxfords, his pale blue shirt, dark blue tie. He's left his walker behind and is going to try it with just his hand crutch. My mother's in a blue dress, sparkly earrings, heels. My uncle is another matter. He's wearing his old yellow see-through sport shirt, his saggy brown tweed jacket, his run-down shoes, his baggy brown pants.

A man named Howard will give us the tour. He's a volunteer and member of the University of Washington Retirement Association—a trim, impeccably neat man with white, short-cropped hair, a bright red sweater, dress pants, brown loafers with tassels. We sit in the lobby while he gives us a general introduction. Howard begins with the history of University House. I think the name has a nice ring. My parents have been given a preferred place on the waiting list, Howard explains, because my father is a college professor emeritus.

Suddenly my father begins to sneeze. Large, bellowing sneezes. "*Excuse* me. I must be allergic to something," he says after every sneeze. It goes on and on. Howard cannot continue. Finally he shuts his eyes, puts down his folder. "Why don't we have the tour now?" he says, getting up.

Given half a chance, I choose catastrophe every time. So now I'm thinking that my father is profoundly allergic to something in this place: the carpet, the paint, the cleaning supplies, the very air. But soon I push that thought out of my mind and look to my father, who has laid his hand crutch on the floor beside the chair, which he is now struggling to get out of. He rocks back and forth, trying to get some leverage, but the chair is too low. My husband takes one elbow and my uncle the other, and get my father to his feet. When Howard picks up the folder

I see him writing something down. We are looking this place over, but he is also looking us over.

In the minus column:
Husband (Allergies and God-knows-what. Handicap significant)
Brother (Uncommunicative. Difficult?)
In the plus column:
Wife (well turned out.)

But then Howard quells his irritation and retrieves his greeter's smile. "Well. Let's start with the apartment. I can show you the rest later." So we head toward the elevators and to an apartment that's in the configuration my parents want: two bedrooms, one on either side of the living room, each bedroom with its own bath. One side for my parents, one for my uncle. My father is leaning heavily on his hand crutch by now, and my mother has taken his other arm.

The elevator doors open to the second floor, and we go down the hall to the appointed door. The woman is away for the holidays and has consented to let her apartment be shown. Howard knocks. No answer, of course. "Let's go in," he says and turns the master key and opens the door.

A woman shrieks and rushes into the living room, clutching her robe to her chest. She stands there in her flowered robe, her pale, bare legs, bare feet.

"Oh," Howard gasps. "Oh my, no. I'm so sorry. This apartment was supposed to be available for viewing. There has been a terrible mistake. You were supposed to be away."

"I came home early. I just got in last night. It's all right," she says shakily. "But you'll have to excuse me. I'm not dressed to receive visitors."

"Oh no. Of course not. I'm so sorry." Howard backs up and turns away. The woman closes the door, and we can hear the lock click into place. Howard's sense of decorum has been shattered. "Just a moment," he says. His mouth is a grim line of determination. "Obviously we'll have to find another apartment. I'll be right back. So many people coming and going these days," he says over his shoulder. So he leaves us standing on the second floor hall back by the elevator while he dashes off to phone the office. My father leans against the wall. "I wish I could sit down," he says.

But soon the elevator doors snap open, and there is Howard, back in a flash, with his red holiday sweater, his pinched smile, his clipboard, two rosy spots high on his cheekbones, a sheen across his forehead. He's gathered his dignity, and the official tone is back in his voice.

"Well. Everything's all right now. There's another apartment we can view. You'll just have to forgive if things aren't quite in order. The resident is getting ready to move out. But you'll be able to get a good idea of the layout, anyway. We have to go up to the fourth floor now."

This apartment isn't on anybody's A-list for prospective residents, but it's what's at hand at the moment, and the resident is willing. And it would be available sometime next month. "It might be just what you're looking for. It has two large bedrooms and two baths, kitchenette, dishwasher, washer and dryer."

Yes, oh yes, I think, let it be a miracle apartment. Let it be everything they ever wanted. Let it be full of sun and light and all good things. Let them see themselves right here. I think of the winters, the ice, the snow, those terrible steps. But safety is so close at hand. Please, please, please, let it be, let this be the one. I cross myself secretly, my hand at my throat, and it's my husband who is the Catholic in the family.

Poor Howard. He just stands at that brass knocker, confident as ever. *Tap tap tap.* A woman shouts, "Come *ih-un*, it's unlocked." So Howard swings the door open and then steps back so fast he almost trips over my father's hand crutch. A woman so large she has literally melted into her wheelchair is sitting in the middle of what should be the living room, but is unidentifiable as it is. She is waving grandly. "Come in, come in!" she says again, as though she had been expecting us all along. The gray carpet is ringed with huge, arcing black smudges from the wheelchair.

The whole apartment has been turned into shelves. Shelves full of pills of all kinds, enormous bottles of vitamins and herbs and potions lining every wall. We peek into the bathroom. There is no bathtub anymore, no shower. Every square inch of wall space holds shelves full of giant bottles of pills. The apartment is a pharmaceutical warehouse.

"Well." Howard turns to us for the next line but we are bereft of speech. "Well," he says. "Well."

"Look around all you want," the woman says, scooting herself forward. "Don't be shy." She turns to look at a tall, gaunt man with a long, dark ponytail, who has mysteriously appeared from one of the rooms, carrying a large cardboard box. It's a scene out of a Hitchcock movie. He doesn't acknowledge us or catch our gaze.

"Just make yourself at home now," she says, inching forward on little pink feet in little pink slippers. Those feet could never support a body like that. No wonder she was in a wheelchair. Had she ever had company? Had she ever come out of her room? Her hair lay in stringy brown strands across her scalp. "We could have *tea*! Do you want tea?"

"Oh no no," Howard says, backing up again. "Thank you, no." The thought clearly appalls him. He vaguely points to the rooms that would have been bedrooms and bathrooms in an ordinary life, then stumbles out of the apartment, as we trail behind.

It's such a dark thing to see. A mind fallen in on itself. The batty old lady in the house condemned, or living with a thousand cats, or pulling a grocery cart of belongings down the street talking to herself—and here she is in apartment 426. The soul of old age, in all its appalling eccentricity and hypochondria right there in the middle of the day. All the shelves full of pills for this and pills for that, for all the things you could name and all the things you couldn't. A shiver crawls up my neck. Had no one seen this? It's so shocking there is no way to make it comic.

Even later, I cannot make this a funny scene, and that has always been my role in our family. All those pills to fend off death, whether it was just around the corner, or years away, it was all the same—a turning from life toward some bleak and lightless place. In that sunless apartment the shadow of death hovered over everything. I remembered later that all the curtains were drawn.

I wondered how she'd ever passed the mental test. Or did she get that way suddenly, in a deepening rush right behind their backs? Well, she would be moving out soon. I wondered if she was being evicted. If she were, Howard didn't know about it. Of course the apartment should never have been shown. It was a mixup of the most egregious kind.

In old age, the hold to decorousness is a hold to a full moon waning. In the years to come I would see it over and over. The secret life of the body's indiscretions disguised with sweet talcum, a spritz of White Shoulders or Evening in Paris, a little rouge, a honey-colored wig, the month's supply of Depends stacked in the bottom of the closet, the little pad for emergencies carried in a clutch purse perfectly matching the shoes. The wool pleated skirt and matching wool sweater, the no-nonsense but elegant Italian loafers for dinner.

I could not let it go. That room full of darkness making a mockery of the chandelier in the lobby, the French club, the glass sculptures. And so you wonder what other dark and unspeakable things go on behind all those closed doors up and down every hallway. Ah, the darker secrets—the smell and touch of them when we hunker down with our terrors and lost loves, and abandoned hopes, and watch how life bends us if it does not break us and remember how we thought it would never happen to us.

But soon we are back on the tour. Howard has recovered sufficiently to show us the *piece de resistance*, the Gallery—with the grand piano, the brocade chairs and love seats, the teak table with the chess set carved from stone, the bookshelves with the *Wall Street Journal*, the *New York Times*, the well-stocked library, and the Dale Chihuly glass sculpture collection. This would make up for everything. "Isn't this just spectacular?" he says as his arm takes in the whole room. He did not tell us that it was also the setting for the memorial services held at regular intervals, announced with dignity in flyers put up in the elevators. What could you expect? The average age here is eighty-four.

Then Howard draws us over to one particular Chihuly installation. "To have such beauty right here . . . ," he trails off. His eyes mist over. He has moved himself to tears. It is beautiful. I thought of Georgia O'Keeffe's flowers. Petals unfolding. Life beginning. Oysters in their secrets lying on the ocean floor, catching the light filtering down from the sun.

Macchia Set

Yellow/Blue

1980

on loan

It's at least a yard wide, a yard long, sitting in its radiant, teakwood case.

But my uncle is having none of it. Not the baby grand or the chandelier or the books and certainly not the Chihuly glass sculptures. He leans over and looks in close. "Did the inmates make this in craft class?" he asks. It's an appalling thing to say. Howard rolls his eyes, says something like "*humph*," and throws up his hands.

"*Henry*," my mother hisses. I want to smack him. You bad boy. You bad bad boy. You behave. You're lucky to be here. Don't you know that? You're lucky they took you in. You're lucky they love so much.

I know what it is. He's just afraid. He's seen it for himself. Every fear of old age rising up before him in that sunless apartment. No wonder he called them *inmates*. The idea of a move had terrified him long before this disastrous visit. And so he thought of every possible danger awaiting them: volcanic eruptions, earthquakes, floods. He'd been through the Mount Saint Helens eruption, Florida hurricanes, and a tornado or two, and knew something about natural disasters. He did not mention the more likely retirement community horrors such as fires, food poisoning, viruses sweeping the halls, residents falling like trees in an ice storm and no way out.

But my uncle's fears have turned to bitterness and the sense that a retirement community is a prison and that he is going to jail. Yet there he is. My parents will take him with them wherever they go, like a child forever on the edge of being lost. He has lived with them close to twenty years and now they will come to this place, or some such place, where they will live out the rest of their lives. He'll have his own bedroom and walk-in closet, his own bathroom. Everything as it was, and nothing as it would ever be again.

Then Howard is herding us back to the elevator. My father can't walk any farther, and nobody wants that to show. My parents are past seeing anything anyway. Thank you, we say hurriedly and make our way down the elevator and out of the lobby, with no turning back to notice the rows of red and white poinsettias lining the presidential staircase into the lobby or the chandelier, or the art on the walls, or the elegant fir tree in the corner decorated in silver and pink.

It's a blessing that my parents remember little of that visit, and only remark with humor and amazement once or twice over the crazy old lady in the room full of pills. But as it turns out, none of them really saw a thing. They were so worried about being rejected as too old, too infirm, and so fearful of the future. I know they will never move here now. They will fall down in the winter, or the spring, or the summer. They will fall down and die and I won't be able to save them.

Moving Mom and Dad and Uncle Henry

While we wait for an apartment at University House to open up for the three of them, our firstborn son is planning a wedding. Christopher Edward is getting married. It's the middle of the summer, and relatives on both sides are beginning to assemble. Robb and Courtney will stand up with their brother, of course. But I have no brothers or sisters, nieces or nephews, aunts or uncles, save Uncle Henry. My much-loved cousin, Carol, is coming with her husband and son. And that's it. And my parents, who don't think they are fit to travel.

"But we could do just what we did at Christmas," I say. "Ed could come and get you and fly you over."

"That's a thought," my mother says, which is always her understated way of saying not a chance.

"But you *have* to be there," I say. It comes out sharper than I intended, and my mother blinks. But I keep on. "We're not doing this without you. There are so few of us. Chris would be so sad." Their faces grow tight. My uncle says, "Whatever you do, Homer." If I can't even get them over for Chris's wedding, their first grandchild's wedding, I could never get them to leave this house and come to live in Seattle.

But miraculously, reluctantly, they agree. So, my husband will fly to Spokane, pick them up in a rental car, drive them to the airport, reserve two wheelchairs, one for my father, of course, and now one for my uncle. He'll push them both while my mother trails behind. Two identical-looking men in wheelchairs with canes across their laps. Then they'll all fly to Seattle, where they'll stay with us the night before the wedding. We're hosting the rehearsal dinner, so they'll get to be there for that too. The next morning we'll all pack up and ride the ferry across the Sound, check into a hotel in Silverdale, a few miles from the wedding the next day. Then when it's over we'll do it all again in reverse. But they will be there.

We are home no more than ten minutes when I hear a loud smack and turn the corner to see my uncle lying face down in the doorway. He has tripped over the door sill and fallen straight on his face. He has bruised his knee and his cheek and his glasses are bent. But we get him up and walking around, and astonishingly, he is intact. My husband straightens Uncle Henry's glasses without breaking the frames, and the mark on his cheek fades within minutes. But at least for now there will be no stairs to climb, no far places to fall. No ice or darkness, or cold. But it is an omen.

In the night my father falls out of bed. He was either getting up to use the bathroom or getting back into bed. He is sprawled on the floor and can't quite remember how he got there. Now my mother is tapping on our door, which we have left ajar, like we did when the kids were little. "Homer fell," she says shakily. "Can you help get him back into bed? I don't think he hurt himself."

Two down, one to go, I think darkly. I will never keep them safe, neither here nor there. But the thought vanishes in a flicker. Tomorrow is going to be a big day. Tomorrow is a wedding. Tomorrow will be full of bright and sacred things.

We sit under a white, billowy canopy that has turned the bride's family's backyard into a fairyland. The sun shines on Liberty Bay, and the Olympics beyond. The flowers shimmer in the breeze. Robb and Courtney stand on either side of the bridal couple. I want to cry. It is all too much, my son getting married, all my children together in that moment, Maureen, the beautiful bride, standing under the festooned archway, the sun shining down on them, blessing them. My father sits beside me in a wheelchair.

The bride and groom exchange their vows:

"Now, for the two of you
Waking up in a royal bed by a garret window. . . .
Yes, this is my gift to you. Above ashes
On a bitter, bitter earth. . . .
Two faces in a mirror
Are only forever once, even if unremembered,
So you watch what is, though it fades away,
And are grateful every moment of your being."

I look down at the program for a minute, catch the words from Rilke and think of my father and uncle. "That even between the closest people infinite distances exist . . . which gives them the possibility of always seeing each other as a whole and before an immense sky." It's what my father could never quite understand and has always feared. Our separateness from him. After all, he has been one half of a whole all his life. That's why he has always feared the Great Divide. I look over at my father and uncle, so alike, even now. They have been called *the twins* their whole life, identical to the last. I wonder just then how my uncle will survive without my father. Though my uncle was firstborn by a minute, it's clear who's going first.

At the reception, my father and uncle are jovial, make jokes, enjoy talking to people stopping by. They are both in their Sunday best, boutonnieres on their lapels. My uncle, who is wearing his good gray suit, is as charming as he ever was. My father, who is always charming, is sunlit by the day. His grandson's wedding after all. He tells me later how memories kept washing over him. It's one of his favorite memories and now he tells it again, how he was taking two-year-old Chris to the bathroom at the restaurant and they wander around a little lost and Chris announces to everyone in earshot that "Grandpa doesn't know where the potty is!" It has always comforted him somehow to retrieve memories of our childhood, mine and the kids. Some part of him fears we would grow out of our love for him once we became adults. But now here is his grandson all grown up and getting married and how much, even now, Chris had wanted him here.

My mother's wearing a blue silk dress, spiky heels, blue, shimmery earrings. I hardly recognize her. She's under siege from worries she has not let go of for a moment. My mother has to go to the bathroom. I lead her into the house then out the front door. There are only a few stairs, maybe only six or seven, leading out of the house to the guesthouse where we will use the bathroom. But there is no railing and my mother is wearing heels. I do not take her arm. I am thinking of a thousand other things, all the people I have yet to greet, my obligations as mother of the groom. The happy couple. I have yet to speak to my sister-in-law and her family. I am thinking of everything but this: those six concrete stairs with no railing. When I remember my mother beside me, I turn and she is gone.

"Mom?" I say, and whirl around. There she is, making no sound, lying face down in the rosebushes. She does not move. She has not made a sound the whole time. She has not cried out, or said *oh no*. Her face has disappeared into the roses, the rosebushes that have saved her, cushioned her fall. My husband's niece's husband rushes over, takes charge. I don't know where my husband or sons are. Now he's gently extricating her from the thorns, helps her to stand up, checks her arms and legs, looks into her eyes. The thorns have cut her legs, torn her stockings. "I'm all right," she says. But she's not. She doesn't ask to sit down or for a glass of water or anything. She just stands there completely silent because there is no way she could have fallen just like that. She has to be the one who is still standing;

there is no other. She doesn't know yet that there are other people now who can catch her. Yet I have let her fall.

But I'm here now, standing right there beside her. I get her sitting down, bring her water anyway, then excuse myself. My daughter is sobbing in the bride's dressing room. She has seen everything. She is shattered and so am I. I should have taken her arm. It was only six steps. I didn't remember there was no railing, though it was the first thing I should have noticed. She could have pitched forward and struck her head on the concrete stairs going down, broken her arm, her hip, her neck. But she had turned quick as a wink and floated down into the rose-bushes. It's a miracle. It's the most terrible thing I have ever seen. I look up at the sky and forget for the moment how stupid it was to think I could keep them safe.

So we all thank our good fortune that she could fall so far without hurt, and try to go on. After all, it's a wedding we're celebrating. But underneath the clothes, and this is the part my mother tells no one until later, the bruises are already beginning to flower. And one place on her shin has been bruised to the bone, and a week later back home, she's still dabbing it with hydrogen peroxide, which only cauterizes the blood vessels needed for healing. She will ignore it until infection sets in so deeply a virtual crater develops on her shin. "We'll have to hospitalize you," they say in the ER where she finally takes herself after my father insists. He rarely takes charge of anything these days. But he does now.

"You need a course of IV antibiotics," the ER doctor tells her. "That infection has gone all the way to the bone. Actually, you really should be in the hospital."

This she cannot, will not, do. I can see her sitting on the edge of the examining table, panic rising in her throat so that for a moment she cannot speak. I can see the set of her mouth, hear the way her voice drops when she will not be moved. Finally she says, "No, I can't do that. Who would take care of my husband?" The thought frightens us all. Who *would* take care of him? Not my uncle. He needs some taking care of himself. We did not know of people you can call, who come in and do more or less what she has always done.

"All right then," the doctor says, "but only if you come in every day for IV antibiotics." He wants her to know how serious this is, and she almost does.

Eventually, after several months, her "wound," as she calls it, heals, but it leaves a permanent mark. Whenever I look at her leg, I see her lying face down in the rosebushes. And several years down the road it is in just that place where a blood clot flowers into bloom, and then she goes to the hospital for sure. But by then there is no one else to worry about. So they all fell down. Ashes to ashes, dust to dust. They seemed perpetually to walk in harm's way. There were so many ways to fall.

And thus begin my falling dreams. It's the same dream over and over, with slight variations. My father is in a hotel lobby, swinging a golf club, warming up for the trip to the top floor of the hotel. He's on his way someplace else and is only staying over. There's a rockery surrounding a little waterfall in the lobby. It's like a sand trap or a waterhole, and one of the hazards of the game. But he's standing too close, and when he swings the club he falls face down onto the rocks. He lies so still I think he's dead, but I wake up before I can tell for sure. Even in the first waking of the day the dream loses none of its poignancy or dread. I spend a long morning trying to figure it out. He's in a hotel, so he's waiting to go from one place to another. He's someplace in between. He's brought along his golf clubs so he's not afraid. He knows where he's going. He's going to the top floor.

On another night it's my mother who falls. We're both standing by the signal light, waiting to cross the street. She takes a step and catches her heel on the curb and begins to fall. My father sees this from the other side of the street and dashes out into the traffic to save her. I reach out just before her head hits the ground, but my hands are too far away. Then I look up and see that my father has disappeared into the flow of cars rushing by. It's all in slow motion so it seems like I can catch them both. So I stand there on the curb with my arms open as wide and far as I can, as they slip just out of reach.

My uncle is wearing his brown jacket, his see-through yellow shirt, his dreaming clothes. He's staggering across our back lawn because he has forgotten his cane. Then he starts to fall forward and plunges down the slope into the gulley, into the blackberry bushes. He's struggling to get up, but the brambles are tearing him apart. I can see his hands and face bleeding from here. He begins to moan. "Don't move. Don't move. I'm coming!" I shout, and scramble down the embankment. But when I get to the bottom of the gulley he is gone. The blackberry bushes are as impenetrable as ever, and as undisturbed.

The falling dreams become as much a refrain these days as the starving dreams, though I have long ago made peace with them. I know what they mean. They are always the same. I have a little girl baby whom I've somehow forgotten about. She's hungry and wet and I have no food, no diapers, no clothes. Or my little blue parakeet from childhood, whom I thought had died long ago, but who has been alive all this time, without food or water for years and years. But then there it is, all feathers and bone. Her beak opens and closes. She pecks around in her empty food dish, bobs her head in the water dish gone dry.

These dreams come if I have not been writing. It's easy to see who's starving who. But the falling dreams are something else. They are pure terror and grief. To see the slow-motion fall into death through my outstretched hands is unbearable in the dream and unbearable as I carry it shuddering into the day.

There are fewer ways to fall in a retirement community than in a house of stairs. So when the phone call finally comes, pulled across the miles by incantations, potions, and spells, it seems nothing short of yet another miracle. We knew it would be sudden when it came. Let's say you're next on the list and a vacancy appears. You have forty-eight hours to take it or leave it. My parents have already turned it down two times, and will not get another chance. They would plummet to the bottom of a waiting list now over two hundred names long, which they would never outlive, or else they would be so far gone they would never pass the entrance exam.

In the third week of August an apartment at University House that matches their specifications—two bedrooms, one on either side of the living room, two bathrooms—suddenly opens up. A vacancy usually means only one thing. The only way people leave this place is to go quietly on a gurney out the side door, in an ambulance off to the ER, or carted off to a nursing home for good. Were there no vacant apartments that had not been visited by death? To move to such a place, you had to stop yourself from thinking about it. No one ever admitted to seeing, in an inadvertent, careless glance, how the angel of death sometimes hovers over the Dale Chihuly glass, the chandelier, the baby grand, or to seeing that dark flicker across your eyes, or the sudden shadow that brushes against your cheek. But all this beauty tells something else—that after virtually all has been said and done, this precious, brief time of life is worthy of such things.

But it is a house divided.

My uncle: "I'm not ready to move. I can't possibly move."

My mother: "All our stuff. Where would it go?"

My father: "Well we've got to move."

My uncle: "They have earthquakes in Seattle."

My father: "Oh, not really."

My uncle: "Mount Rainier might erupt. Lava could reach Seattle."

My father: "No it couldn't. Not really."

My uncle: "It rains all the time."

My father: "No it doesn't. Ice and snow are harder than rain."

My uncle: "What about my doctors?"

My father: "You can get new ones. They have good doctors in Seattle."

My mother: "All the stuff in the garage and the basement. Where will it all go?"

My father: "We don't need all that stuff anyway. We'll just sell it."

My mother: "But who would buy it?"

My father: "We'll give it away if we have to, because we're going."

My mother: "Well we'll just have to stay here till we croak."

• • •

Aunt Bee isn't her real name, of course. But it gives her a motherly, you-can-trust-me kind of image. She's a large woman with graying brown hair, sensible sandals, a cotton house dress, big, pale pink-framed glasses. She will help my parents get from one place to the other. She will make the three floors of stuff go away. I didn't know there were people who did such things. My son, Chris, doesn't like her from the start, thinks she's a con artist, the way she patronizes my parents, the way her eyes sweep the room as she talks, sizing everything up. The accoutrements of my parents' life for the last thirty-five years are in her tally now: what to grab for herself to sell, what to put in the estate sale, or recycle to the next one. "You just let Aunt Bee handle everything," she says, patting my father's hand.

After the four of us—Chris and Courtney and Maureen, our brand-new daughter-in-law, and I—have triaged and sorted and boxed everything up, put green dots on the things to go, and red dots on the things to stay, Aunt Bee will hold a three-day estate sale after we are gone, completely and forever gone. She'll make the rest, all the things nobody wanted, go away. It's all right, no matter what Aunt Bee is up to. Because she will do what my mother has wanted. She will make everything go away. And the house will be empty of all that has been. It will be painted and recarpeted, and then some lovely family with easy financing and a bunch of kids will buy it and think it's a miracle house, a blessing house.

Our little crew of four sorts through and packs up everything in that three-story house in less than a week. Robb's in Tokyo teaching English, and Ed's in Seattle in the first days of his new job as athletic director at Lakeside School, an elite private prep school in north Seattle. After years of coaching and teaching in the hurly-burly of the public school system, Ed had retired. He was barely fifty. But after four months off the job in a season of ninety days of rain without ceasing, he began looking at the want ads. He could sell lumber at a lumber yard. He could measure and cut wood. After all, he'd built our house. Ed has always been oblivious to status or class. He came from a blue-collar family. His mother did not finish high school and though his father wanted to go to college and become an engineer, he didn't have the money. So he worked for Burlington Northern Railroad repairing boxcars. Ed was the first one in his family to go to college.

Now he's gone back to work in this new job at a private school with tuition that costs more than a lot of colleges. But to him, kids are kids and every one of them needs a little help now and then.

Back in the old public school days, things often went something like this: We're all having dinner in the little kitchen in our old house by the freeway, and I'm trying to squeeze in a bit of adult conversation as the kids chatter on. I start things off.

"How was your day?" I ask Ed.

"Okay."

"Anything interesting happen?"

"No, not really," he says.

And so it goes. Though halfway through dinner he gets up, takes his plate to the sink, and says, "You know I'm going to swing by the ER and get my shoulder checked out. I think I might have dislocated it."

I jump up. "Are you all right? What happened?"

"Oh, at lunch this kid was high on something and went after another kid with a tire iron. I think I screwed up my shoulder when I wrestled him down."

"I should drive you."

"Hey, I got home, didn't I? I'll be fine. No point in taking all the kids to sit in the ER."

Now he'll begin work at Bill Gates's alma mater. He'll love this job above all others. He'll love the humanity and sense of social justice and environmental responsibility that is at the heart of the mission of this school. He'll love the kids as always. But here there will be no tire irons in the lunch room. Some things will change. Others will remain the same.

If Robb hadn't been in Japan and my husband in Seattle, everyone I loved would have been in that house for the last time, going through these last things together. But in such a move, so careless and so fast, you have to go through everything as best you can before you decide to keep it or throw it away. The blessing and the curse is what you find in the process.

Found: A metal box belonging to my grandfather Lisle, my mother's father, who lived with us along with my grandmother, during the last year of his life, when he was dying of heart failure. It was the year we switched our bedrooms around. I moved down to the basement, where my parents fixed up a room for me. They took apart the bunk beds I'd had in my room upstairs next to theirs, and made them into two single beds, for sleepovers, in the room downstairs. My parents managed to fit themselves into my little bedroom upstairs, which held their double bed and little more, and my grandparents took the master bedroom, which was big enough to accommodate a hospital bed so my grandfather could sleep propped up for the night. The oxygen delivery truck came every Tuesday and pronounced to the neighbors that someone in that house was ill. Someone in that house was dying.

In that metal box we find a statement of bankruptcy, a narrative of pure loss without recovery or transcendence. My grandfather had invested in some timberland in Oregon, after he'd moved out West, and had been cheated out of all his investment money. He sold real estate then, and his failing heart permitted him no ease in getting in and out of cars, or taking clients up and down stairs and down all those blocks to the houses he never sold. Eventually my grandparents could not pay their bills, and so they moved from Walla Walla to our first house, a little two-bedroom house in Spokane the summer I was twelve. My age of knowing.

How humiliated my grandfather must have been to move in with us then, how he must have hoped that a last, most desperate measure—a valve-replacement surgery—would restore his health, let them move out, be on their own again. He knew what a strain my grandmother was. But of course he died, and she lived on with my parents until her own death at ninety-three. My mother's parents: Lisle and Edna Piper. I loved him and not her, though she's the one who stayed behind.

But my father loved my grandfather Lisle too. He called him Dad. He did things with his father-in-law he had never done with his own father. My grandfather was a patient, gentle teacher, and he taught my father many things. He taught him how to do things with tools; he taught him to shoot, and when they went hunting together my father shot his first and only deer.

The night my grandfather died, three days after heart surgery to fix what could not be fixed, my father stayed with him all through the night until he died early the next morning. I had seen my grandfather only once after he went to the hospital, the second night after surgery, when my parents let me go with them to the hospital. I did not say goodbye or I love you, or any such thing. I only remember sitting wordlessly in a chair beside the bed, staring at his bare chest. It was painted orange up to his chin. I don't remember any bandages or tubes. Just that orange paint everywhere and how scared I was trying to think of something to say.

We go too fast through those papers in the metal box to feel the sting in our prying eyes. There is my grandparents' wedding license, the one they'd hidden for years, the one that showed the date of their marriage seven months before my mother's supposed premature birth. Since she weighed in at over eight pounds, it was something to think about. So Grape had gotten him the only way she could. That was the only way my mother and father had to explain why this gentle, heroic man would marry a woman like my humorless grandmother. My parents had a theory about my grandmother: that in every large family, one child becomes, in the pecking order, the one chick pecked on and bloodied and pushed out of the flock. I remember it now. The only sympathetic memory I have of her in all those years. At my grandfather's funeral, she walked up to his coffin to say goodbye. She took off her white glove and patted his face. "Oh, how I will miss you," she cried.

My grandmother had a soprano voice so resonant and clear my mother claims she could have sung opera professionally, if only she'd had the training and a way to travel to New York—a voice that in her day, was good for church solos and little else. My voice never had the resonance of my grandmother's, but that we both sang soprano was a little similarity I could claim, if I had not spent most of my life looking for all the ways we were different.

All the beauty and grace she was ever going to have was distilled into that one, solitary gift. It must have been what my grandfather had fallen in love with. Or maybe something else, as my parents had always thought, given my mother's "premature" birth. This little metal box holds the fragments of their lives that had not caught in the net of memory or photograph. All families must have such stories of lives that could have been and were not, stories recovered by chance that bring the gift of insight and grief.

In the process of letting go, my mother has culled everything down to three. My mother has always been a minimalist, and this is no grief to her. Three spoons, three forks, three knives, three cups, plates, glasses, a couple of pots and pans. She will give up cooking. The burden of the house and its contents has weighed on her for so long it's a lark, this letting go. Do you want this? No. That? No. After the weight of things for so long, she must have felt like flying. Goodbye to the snow on the roof and the drainpipes clogged with leaves, goodbye to the lawn and the sprinklers, goodbye to the driveway packed with snow, goodbye to the basement with a hundred boxes, goodbye to the garage and the lawnmower and edger and garden hoses and cans of paint and paint thinner and brushes.

In the beginning, my mother insisted that we find room in the new apartment for her china cabinet, the only household possession she had ever loved, and her only wavering. It will now go to me.

"I'm just safekeeping it for you," I say. I want her to have the one thing she loves, but there is no room where she's going.

"We want it to stay in the family," my father says. He means that it's mine now. I'm not safekeeping it. It's never going back. When I was growing up, our family had moved so many times my mother had learned not to become attached to anything. I, on the other hand, always wanted to take everything I had. But she traveled light. The only thing she ever needed for her travels was my father.

My mother's makeup has lain untouched in her bathroom drawer since the morning of my father's stroke. It was always a great pleasure for her, the ritual, the transformation. But she has no time for such things now and has me throw it all out.

"But maybe you'll want to pick it up again," I say. She just looks at me. All her time is spent saving my father now. She's too weary for makeup. It's an effacement so absolute I know if I am saving anyone by this move, I am saving her.

My father wants to take all his books. He doesn't care about anything else. "We won't have room for these," my mother says. "We're only taking one little bookcase." We don't point out that he did not read books anymore, as far as we could tell, and his days of research are gone forever. So we cull them as best we can and put the precious ones in boxes we will store somewhere on our own. I want to take all his books too. The record of his thinking cannot be left behind.

My uncle is going to donate his thousand books to the Whitworth College library, but of course he doesn't get around to doing this until the very last day. "*Please please please* don't wait until the last minute for things, Uncle Henry. I'll have so much else to do I can't be driving you all over town." But of course that's just what he does. He waits until the very last day to sort through and then donate his books; sell his car, which he has not driven in five years; fill his prescriptions at the medical clinic forty-five minutes away on the other side of town; close out his bank accounts; go through ten years of unopened mail; pack his suitcase.

Of course, I'm mad as hell driving from the medical clinic across town to the bank the afternoon before the big move. And so when my uncle mentions, apropos of nothing, the day his father died, I say, "So. Uncle Henry, tell me how your father died again." It's wicked and I know it. Grandfather James, whom I hardly knew.

"Oh," he says, gathering the images before him. "He was out for a walk and keeled over just like that." He has said it so ingenuously I knew he didn't know what had really happened. It's one of the more interesting of our family secrets, one that has been kept from him all these years. But I am so angry with him I say, "Really. I'd always heard he died in a slightly *different* way."

"No, he just keeled over during a walk."

"Really? Just like that."

"Yes, it was just like that." My uncle says it even now, with a kind of tender and innocent astonishment, as though he couldn't quite believe it yet himself.

It was my father who told me the story of how my uncle had violently opposed his father's marriage to Lillian in the year after their mother, Alfreda, died. How Henry had tried to stop their marriage, had in fact rushed after them as they made their way from Michigan, where James had his church since the boys were teenagers—to Florida, where they were to be married. It dishonored his mother's memory. It shamed his father some way. It was obscene. "She's no older than *I* am," he said over and over. He was right. Lillian and the twins were thirty-three. He could not say the name of his father's new wife. He could not say *Lillian.* "She was just waiting in the wings to grab him." Lillian was a nurse, and one of those who helped care for Alfreda in her last days, so I guess my uncle was right in a small way and wrong in a bigger one.

Before his marriage to Lillian, my grandfather had been director of all the Free Methodist churches in the state of Michigan. He was in the process of building a new, bigger church when Alfreda died. But church leaders disapproved of the marriage so strongly they removed him from his large Battle Creek Free Methodist Church and sent him to a much smaller, out-of-the-way church in the countryside. So for love, James and Lillian became outcasts of the universe. And Alfreda would never know the astonishing way her husband would die.

My father had given his blessing to his father's new marriage right from the start, glad that Lillian had given his father such happiness. Because James had told my father a secret within a secret: Alfreda had kept her marriage to James unconsummated for that first, long year, when he thought he would go crazy with wanting her. And then later when the twins were born, she kept them in the bedroom with them for the first three years. And so for a very long time there was no intimacy, and very little after.

Alfreda had been engaged before and had watched her first fiancé drown. Afterward she had said, *I will never smile again*, or so it has been recorded in memory down through the years. And the rest of what I know came to me from my father's cousin, the family historian.

My father's cousin has always wanted to know who begat who. He would leave interpretation to others. All these mysteries neither of us could solve as we both looked through the fog of years, now that so many of the beloved are gone. I was trying to see the figure in the carpet. I was trying to see the long arc of their lives in spite of what must have seemed the sad, dark end of it. A thing whole and complete has a beauty of its own, even when the things apart are too terrible to say.

Then my cousin added: "I think you'll find this interesting." And I noticed he'd sent an attachment.

It was the front page of the *Atlanta Constitution*, May 1, 1909: "Victims of Drowning in Waters of Lakewood." Under that headline are two pictures. One of them is of my grandmother Alfreda. The other is her fiancé, William Withrow. But it was William and his sister, Pearl, who drowned, not Alfreda.

Brother dies in vain attempt to save sister. William and Pearl Withrow find a watery grave. . . . None could tell why the boat capsized and the real reason will probably go down as another in the long list of mysteries surrounding this ill-fated lake.

But that headline tells a certain truth. Alfreda was a victim of that drowning also, as she brought that dark sorrow into her marriage to my grandfather and to her twin boys.

Once the boat flipped over, she'd gone under fast, her skirts weighing her down, but she'd pushed through the dark green water with her strong, swimmer's legs, to see William swim away from her and toward his sister, Pearl, to see her grasp his neck and pull him down, no thrashing to the surface for a second try. She saw the rush of water knit itself back again, still as glass. When the other boats reached Alfreda, she'd called out to leave her and save the others. She'd stayed like that, hugging the boat for over an hour, refusing rescue until it was clear even to her that they were gone. It was the first of May.

As they carried Alfreda off the dock, she looked back one more time to that place in the water where the boats now circled, so still, so dark. How could he be so suddenly gone? That night she lay numb and disbelieving in her board-inghouse room, while thunder cracked against the house and the wind blew the curtains and someone came in—but who?—to shut the window. She lay with her head in the pillow and tried to sleep, but every time she closed her eyes, she saw him floating over the bottom in that green, murky water, his arms outstretched in astonishment. She did not see Pearl anywhere. It was better to keep her eyes open. So she watched the lightning flash across the sky as Will lay at the bottom of the lake, and she knew her prayers had gone unanswered. When the lightning shattered the sky, she wondered what goodness ruled the universe now.

They'd spread the tablecloth on the grassy hill above the beach, where they'd gone for a picnic—the bowl of fried chicken covered with a white linen napkin, and potato salad and cucumber pickles, fresh bread, and fruit. There would have been chocolate, of course. Pearl would have brought it from the candy store where she worked.

And the next day the trespass of her picture in the paper, her life so suddenly laid open for all to see, how she was carried off, half out of her mind. She was twenty-one. Then the violence of the hooks and barbed wire and dynamite to bring the bodies up. And the taste of the day bitter on her tongue forever after, and the plums, where were the plums? Who had eaten the plums?

It wouldn't have been until after the note inside the green bottle had been found floating near shore that she would have remembered how he'd said a prayer before they took to the water, how Pearl had tipped the boat, how he swam to those wild arms. The note was written on memorandum paper and tied with a red ribbon, holding a message dangerous enough to slay the most fearless heart. How smoothly they had slipped down.

To Whom It May Concern: I and my sister have become tired of life and we have decided to die in this way. Withrow

The whole town had read it now. But who would write such a thing? if not him, and it couldn't have been him. Who would say she was not worth living for? She was afraid to shut her eyes because now she saw Pearl tipping the boat and the two going over together and then the boat flipping and suddenly she was underwater, so green and dark, then pushing to the light and air, yes oh yes, life after all and everything to look forward to, but there was Will swimming to Pearl and not to her.

In the newspaper, Alfreda is posed all in white, one hand against her cheek, the other holding a white parasol. She's looking off in the distance. You can see a slight upturn at the corners of her mouth, as though she had to work to tamp down the smile. She's thinking of something she's waiting for. Then her picture in the watch she gave my grandfather before they were married. It was his birthday. She's dressed in gray, looking straight out at the place in the water where last William was. See? I told you I would never smile again.

And so her life became part of the mythology of that murky lake haunted by its history of drownings and suicides and murder. But Will Withrow was the one she loved. My grandfather, James Cunningham, was the one who came after. And Alfreda went unsmiling into the marriage to my grandfather, this woman I never knew, who died ten days after I was born, our only connection my name in her obituary, her only grandchild. Surely this must have explained her resistance to my grandfather. Her closing up to him, when ordinarily you would spend half your life's allotment of rapture in that first wild year, with all the permission in the world now, and such pleasure you could die from it. So it was easy to imagine all the ways life had given something back to my grandfather, with this second, new young wife, with no aversion to sex, though there would never be any children. James and Lillian would have five years before he died.

Lillian would have to tell someone. She couldn't keep a secret like that forever. How long did she wait before she couldn't wait any longer? It was Homer, my father, not Henry, Lillian told. Did it come rushing out or was it measured and composed? She'd have whispered it to my father as they sat by the woodstove in that Michigan kitchen.

Men must secretly fear it. So it's easy to understand all the nervous jokes with the punch line, *but what a way to go*. Only guys tell a joke like that. But to be the woman, to be as close as breathing when it happened. The weight of him, the *dead weight* of the one you loved, would be no joke. This final intimacy would be no laughing matter. James died from love of her. It was one way of looking at it. Was he a heartbeat away from death the whole time? Or was there some sign to tell her to help him slow things down, or to stop them entirely? It would be enough just to have you, if only you would live. The guilt, the final, shattering intimacy—how could this stay a secret, unconfessed? It would be your last and ever after, abiding image of him, that beloved face gone so strangely slack and pale? Would you turn from it if you could?

To rush for your clothes, and then his. He was a minister after all, and some decorum must be followed. Or was it their wedding sheet, kept white and newly starched these five years, that floated down across his face? Who to call when there was no 911, no aid car or fire department, no CPR, no jump-start at hand? Dead was dead in those days and no calling back.

When I was five, my mother said, "Your daddy's sad now because your granddaddy died." We lived in New York then, in an attic. I remember going to the backyard of our house with the attic and saying a little prayer for my father's sadness.

I have one brief memory of my grandfather James. I'm in the kitchen sitting on my grandfather's lap. We're in Michigan for a visit, the only one I can remember. He's wearing a wool sweater and we're sitting by a woodstove in the kitchen. I must have been three or four. I'm a little afraid of him. It's summer and I'm wondering why he has need of a sweater. It makes my bare arms itch. I'm just sitting there stiffly on his lap, trying to see if he really looks like my father and my uncle, and he does. Lillian is somewhere in the background. I remember her long dark hair tied up in a loose bun. I remember her face was smooth, and she wore rimless glasses that caught the light. She was wearing an apron but not a sweater. Now I think of that long hair coming undone, the pins coming out one by one, then all of it coming down in a waterfall of soft, dark hair.

Years later, over fifty years later, Lillian sends a letter to my parents, about her marriage to my grandfather James. It comes out of the blue, prompted by nothing my mother can imagine, except maybe a putting of affairs in order, as Lillian isn't well herself. But there it is, Lillian's letter, beginning in script, then quickly moving to printing. It's a little yellow piece of paper she's lined to help steady her sloping, trembling hand:

Dear Homer and Grace,

I wanted to tell you about J.B. and me. My father went into a TB sanitarium when I was about 5. He died 3 years later. I didn't know my father. My mother used me every way she could. I had trouble loving God. J.B. was the first person to love me. I saw in him what a father could be like. I guess everything is going well for me. Hope all is okay for you.

Love, Lillian

Maybe this is what she wanted my father to know all these years and could not quite put into words until now. Perhaps she was reckoning with her own life, putting certain ghosts to rest. I find it poignant in its simplicity and directness, and ask to keep it. But there it is. The scandal of his marriage to Lillian, his demotion in the church that had been his life. *J.B.* I had never heard him called J.B. Suddenly I have a grandfather. My grandfather who died of love for her.

I search through my own old things to find the Bible my grandfather had given to my father for Christmas when I was two years old, and my father had given to me. My grandfather had written: "from Pop. With heaps and lots of love. I am so glad that you ever came to live with me." His handwriting could have been my father's. I get out my grandfather James's picture again. For the first time I see what a wonderful face he has. Such lovely, kind, and interested, interesting eyes. He's looking out at the world with an expectation of goodness and an offering of it as well. I had rarely given a thought to this grandfather I had hardly known. Now I look at the old photograph and want to put it in a frame on the wall, or prop it on my desk. He looks so like my father, so like the twins, who look nothing like Alfreda.

So it's all right. Running all over town with my uncle on this the last day. It would take as long as it would take. My uncle is saying goodbye to all the things that have kept him safe. His books, his car, his doctors, his bank, his pharmacy. No wonder this reluctance, until the very last minute. We will get through this day after all. And secrets will remain secrets. Why not?

And so we complete my uncle's errands, one by one, and he really does manage to sell his car, donate the books, do his banking and medical clinic business all in one day. The ten years of unopened mail is another thing. For the last decade of his life he'd refused to open it. It grew into slipsliding piles on his desk and on the floor beside and under his bed. Why *didn't* he open his mail? It was a question to be asked. "Why should I open it?" he said. "I already know what's in it."

Now at the end of the day, and it must have been toward nine o'clock, he finally decides to open his mail. "Mom," Chris says to me, "we've got to stop him. He's just stalling anyway. He'll say he can't move to Seattle till he's done it."

So my son goes down to him and says, "Uncle Henry, you don't really have time to go through all that mail now."

"Sure I do."

"Hey, why don't you take a break and see what's on television? I think that building show might be on." *This Old House.* Both my uncle and father love to watch things being built. Their father, who was a master carpenter as well as a minister, would never let the twins go near his tools. He was always afraid they would wreck something, and he didn't have the time or patience to teach them. So neither boy grew up knowing how to do much in that way, though it was my father, the homeowner, who felt this lack most keenly.

"We can just put your letters in these garbage sacks and store them in your filing cabinet." It will get a green dot. It will go.

"Well, okay," my uncle says. He's subdued now and not up to a fight. I couldn't have persuaded him, though my son finally does.

I have no idea how any of them spent that last night, or whether they slept at all. But we decide that on this last day, breakfast should be as familiar as possible, though all the dishes and pans are either packed away or set aside for the estate sale. "They should have their own breakfast just like they always do," my daughter-in-law says. So Chris and Maureen set out to Rosauer's for a vat of oatmeal, slices of toast, and orange juice and coffee. Now it's the last meal in that kitchen, in this house, and no one feels like eating.

And so we wait. We will leave when the moving van arrives, so we can give final instructions. But it gets later and later, and still the wait goes on. My mother is silent and so anxious over what comes next she has removed herself from the scene entirely. My father has settled deeply into himself, watching or not watching television, I can't tell. They will never see this place again. If they ever come back it will be someone else's house. But there is only one way they will come back to this town, and all of us know which way that is.

I go downstairs to check on my uncle. He'd disappeared down the stairs right after breakfast. There is no breakfast cleanup today.

"Uncle Henry?" I call down. He's not gone back to bed as usual, but is standing spread-eagled in the corner against the wall, his hand against the door. "I can't go. I'm not *ready!*"

"But Uncle Henry, the moving van will be here any minute now."

His eyes are wide and his face has gone sweaty and pale. I remember yesterday and how we talked about his father's death. Uncle Henry's chest is going up and down, up and down. "Uncle Henry," I say quietly, and put a hand on his arm. "Let's go sit down a minute." I lead him to his TV chair and pat his arm, turn on the television. "I'll be back," I say, and race upstairs.

Maureen says to me, "You can't wait for the moving van. You've got to get him out of here now or he's going to have a heart attack or a stroke. Just put them in the car and *go.*"

So we change plans at the eleventh hour. Chris and Maureen will stay behind and wait for the movers, then catch up to us when they can. They'll drive my parents' car across the state after us at speeds it had never seen before. Courtney will inherit this car. The Brown Bomber. Big and luxurious, with brown leather upholstery that will aggrieve her sensibilities every day she drives it, though it will get her reliably from here to there. She flew home yesterday because she couldn't take off another day from work, but will be waiting for us when we arrive.

So we put them in the car, my father in the passenger seat, my mother and uncle in the back, and off we go. I watch the city disappear in my rearview mirror. They do not turn and look behind to say goodbye. I put on a CD, a compilation of classical music I hope will take the edge off. I don't know. Anything but this silence, because none of us can think of a single thing to say.

My father stares straight ahead, says nothing. He's saying goodbye to everything now. Goodbye to Rotary, goodbye to politics, goodbye to the college and the church, goodbye to their friends. In truth the attachments to these things have frayed in the years since his stroke. Friends have called less, dropped by even less. It's only what happens. It's all right. He only loves my mother anyway. He only wants her safe. My mother has no abiding attachments either, not to things or people anymore, only to my father. My uncle has attachments to everything. He wants everything to stay the same. I keep glancing back at his frightened eyes in my rearview mirror.

I'm hoping the thrum of the wheels as we flee down the interstate will put my frantic uncle to sleep. If only he could just let go and fall asleep I wouldn't worry so much about the heart attack or stroke he might be having right now on this long stretch of across the desertlike middle of the state, miles from help in either direction. If he would just fall asleep I could ease my watch of him in the rearview mirror and concentrate on the road ahead.

But then the next time I glance back, his head is turned, his mouth is open. He's just sleeping and not dead, I tell myself, as my heartbeat catches in my throat. I check the mirror a few moments later and see that he's turned his head to the other side, closed his mouth. I don't need to stop the car and put a mirror under his nose to tell me he has not died.

It occurs to me now that all of this has been almost more than they can bear. I wonder if they can recover from such a terrible uprooting. Some things cannot be transplanted. Roots do not take hold. Leaves do not push their way up out of the hoary earth to such wintry light. This very well might be more than my beleaguered mother can bear. And my uncle. Can he survive such a thing? Only my father will be all right. He's already loosening his hold upon the earth.

My father is asleep now too. Only my mother and I are awake. She stares straight ahead, unblinking, down the road, wavery in the distance with the summer heat. We do not even bother with small talk. Suddenly it occurs to me, as it has not before, that I am saying goodbye too. Goodbye to my childhood, and the childhood of my children who spent every holiday of their lives in this place. Two weeks at Christmas, two weeks in the summer, and weekends here and there. Goodbye to all the history of that house with its secret passages and hideaways, nooks and crannies, all the Christmas plays written and performed, the night walks in the snow.

My mother asks me to play the CD again. She asks me to play it over and over. *Scheherazade, La Mer, Daphnis and Chloe,* love theme from *Spartacus.* The music wraps her in comfort. It says everything will be all right. Now, for these blessed hours, nothing is required. No decisions to be made, no care to be given. She settles into the music but does not fall asleep, does not even shut her eyes. The terrain of her unspoken fears vanishes into the music. It's like old times. We stop for bathroom breaks, we stop for lunch—but it takes hours longer than it ever did before. In and out of the car, in and out of the bathroom, the restaurant, the bathroom again, canes and walkers, holding arms and hands.

But I will get them those three hundred miles across the mountains to the new and shining life I have made for them. The old is vanishing behind them, the new is somewhere beyond the mountains we can begin to see in the distance. And so we fly across the state, from one life to another.

Life at The House

It's the end of August, 1999, and we have made the move. And so when they walk into their apartment three days later, everything is as it had been before. While they were camped out at our house thirty minutes away, we had set up their apartment exactly the way it had been in their house before. Toilet tissue on the holders, Kleenex by the bed, wastebaskets in every room, laundry detergent, cleaning supplies, paper towels under the sink, their clothes in the drawers and closets, pictures on the wall. When they walk in they are already home. My uncle can't believe we have done such a thing. "I thought there would be cardboard boxes everywhere," he says over and over. After that terrible uprooting, it's exactly what we want them to see: a place full of comfort, safety, love.

We bought a little half-moon table that now sits against the counter between the living room and the kitchen, perfect for two, but it has a leaf that can be extended to accommodate three, if perchance the happy couple have a guest, a single, permanent guest. It was the one logistical thing we couldn't at first figure out. Where would they eat? No room anywhere in the kitchen or living room. They would get their dinner in the dining room, but breakfast and lunch were on their own. But that little table tucked against the counter, with a little leaf you can raise or lower, and the extra straight back chair works just fine for the third person at this table for two.

And I bought them all new beds, with bedding to match—three single beds. Three times I sent those beds back to the store. I was Goldilocks herself, returning to the store for the third time. I could see the salesman roll his eyes. Here she comes again. Those beds were either too hard, or too soft, too low, or too high, before they were at last just right.

Now they are home. They are together in their own place, with their own things. But once they venture outside their door, they enter a new social environment, with its own secret rules and regulations, its own pecking order, gossip mill, a living, breathing organism where octogenarians abound. "The only thing I don't like about this place," my uncle says, though of course he doesn't like anything about this place, "is that the people here are too *old*." And he's right. It is a house of relics. A museum of precious, ancient things. A house where angels hover and the girl who cleans your apartment and tucks you in at night or listens for your breathing while you sleep is an angel too, because death is your neighbor now or the man behind the desk in the lobby who keeps watch all through the night.

Tonight's their first night at University House, and my parents have pleaded with my husband and me to stay for dinner. I remember thinking it was like dropping your kids off at their first summer camp. Please don't go. Stay with us. We don't want to be alone here. Not yet. And so we do.

They seat us at what will always be known as "the big table." It has become prime real estate in that dining room, the preferred table, but my parents don't know this yet. They just know that people here are friendly right from the start. Introductions all around. "Glad you're here, you'll love this place!" and so forth. But when the food is served everybody pretty much turns their attention to their plates. It's just as well. Eating without spilling is not something you take for granted these days. And besides, it's pretty hard to hear across that wide table anyway.

Summer has not yet given way to fall, and the gardens outside the dining room windows and French doors are blooming with every promise of the year.

Long, lush evenings of light still to come, the late-afternoon sun on the last of the August roses, the last brilliance of the year, the garden's last blooming. Orange and blue and violet, pink and yellow, a lushness that makes your heart ache with the coming of fall just a flicker away. We have crossed them over to safety at last. Now there will be no more stairs, no more ice or snow, or falling trees.

Then my father begins to cough. Soon it's more of a choke than a cough, and now he's grabbing at his throat and his face is turning red, and he leans forward and then can make no sound at all. He's looking wildly at no one in particular. Everything is in slow motion. Time has stopped. I sit there stunned into silence. My mother looks down at her plate and shuts her eyes. My uncle's mouth drops. *Help!* he whispers to the air. Then my husband jumps up and wraps his arms around my father from behind. He puts his fists under my father's breastbone and pushes, two snaps, then two snaps again. The piece of meat comes flying out of my father's mouth and lands on the tablecloth in front of him. He gasps, and falls back in his chair. It has happened so fast my mother and I have not moved an inch. Everybody else just keeps on eating. Sweat runs down the side of my father's face. He takes a napkin in his shaky left hand and wipes his face.

"Oh my," my father says. "I'm sorry." He's embarrassed to have made such a scene. "Oh my," he says again.

"Don't worry, dear," the woman on my right says, patting my arm. "This happens all the time. We just call 911."

Max Applebaum doesn't say a word during all of this, but just smiles at my father from across the table with his generous, sad brown eyes. That's okay, he seems to be saying, it's okay. He's new also, and knows how hard it is to make a good first impression. Their first night and already they have distinguished themselves. People had already been expecting them. *The Cunninghams.* One woman and two identical men.

Those nice guys at the fire station down the block have never had so much business. Up 100 percent since University House came along. When you've fallen down and you can't get up, house rules say you must call 911. That September the staff holds a reception for the medics. Everybody comes. Cookies and punch and coffee to say thanks for coming so fast, for being so kind when we fall, for being sure we're all right, for getting us gently back on our feet. "They're just so nice," my mother's new friend Ginny says. "They treat you so nice no matter what's happened to you," which of course is exactly what my parents say a couple of months later when my father collapses on his way to the bathroom. They learn soon enough what that aid car means. If it's parked in front, it means that the rush through the front door to the elevator is the fastest route in and out, when speed is all that matters. But if the aid car is parked on the side street, it means someone has died, and there is no need for rushing anymore.

My mother and father and my uncle have come to the House of Widows. Five to one—women to men. I'm hoping this place is like a large girls' college dorm, with slumber parties, sleepovers, movie nights with just the girls, because it isn't hard to see that my mother will become a widow here too. "Find somewhere for us to go," my father had said. "I want her safe before I die."

Yet for all its decorousness, the current affairs discussion groups, the lectures and concerts, the French club, this is where they lived now, at the edge of the cliff where no one looks down. My parents have come to this new place, where, beautiful though it is, their lives narrow poignantly—for despite the library and the Gallery and the workout room, and the gardens, they mostly stay in their apartment, where they live uneventfully, medically speaking, through that first autumn.

For two precarious years my parents live in Apartment 320 where dinner was the highlight of the day. You get gussied up for dinner. Maybe you bring a bottle of wine for the table. You might even invite a few neighbors over for wine and cheese beforehand. My parents get fixed up too, put on their name tags, ready to greet the world. Here we are. Please love us. Please be our friend. For my mother, going to dinner is an astonishing relief. No more trips to the grocery store, no more trips across icy parking lots, no more bags of groceries to put away, no more thinking of what to eat, what shall we eat? "We don't care," the twins would say, "anything is fine." And my mother would answer, "I can't cook *anything*. I can only cook *something*."

Now every night's a night out. But there are no tables for three. And so the threesome would always conjure a fourth. From the beginning, two women try to stake a claim on that fourth spot. Each has her eye on my uncle, I am sure, though my children find this impossible to believe. He can still strike a handsome pose. He can still be charming, when he wants to. In fact, in the presence of women he becomes transformed—witty, sly, a little flirtatious in his teasing way.

My father gives him no competition on that score any longer. He's quiet, subdued, in a sweet, sad, wearing-out way. He seems content to observe, add a few comments here and there if they are effortless, but mainly he concentrates on his food, which is a wise move, considering all that has gone before. At first my father comes to dinner using his hand crutch, wearing his camel blazer, his name tag for all to see, then after that first hospitalization a couple of months later, a walker, then his "scooter," which he "drives" to the dining room and parks in the coat closet. Then after that, the wheelchair, which my uncle pushes as much to balance himself as to help my mother. That way Uncle Henry can leave his cane behind, which he's always supposed to use and rarely does, because it ruins his image with the ladies.

My parents' first friends are Peggy and Ginny, two women who hate each other, but who love my parents, and are perhaps a little in love with my uncle. Both Peggy and Ginny expect to be the fourth at the dinner table, and rush to beat the other to what soon becomes the coveted fourth spot. After all, there aren't many single men, steady on their feet. And my uncle is still a looker, and enjoys the flirtations of women.

Peggy is the tiniest woman I have ever seen, in a strange and frightening way. She looks as though she'd once been much taller, and her spine had folded in on itself, like an accordion. Peggy, with her tiny little legs and her smoker's lungs and weathered face, rushing to the table, shouting *Wait for me, wait for* me! Ginny is buoyant and easily the largest woman at University House. She speaks with a Southern accent, knows everybody by name, plays gin rummy like a champ, and shares a riotous and outrageous sensibility with my mother, who has been a secret rebel all her life. Ginny pushes her walker at a pretty good clip, even with the accompanying oxygen tank, so it's always a race to see who can reach the dining room first, and that empty fourth spot.

Then Peggy begins calling my mother to "reserve" the fourth spot in advance. It upsets my mother greatly to be disappointing one or the other of them all the time. "Just don't answer the phone," I tell my mother. But this she cannot do, as I cannot, because from now on, phone ringing cannot be ignored. So my mother takes it up with Donna, the dining room supervisor, who understands perfectly, and agrees that some of the time she'll seat my parents at a table for eight, and give them all a break. Then later, with Peggy near tears, they agree that she'll have Tuesday night dinner, and Ginny Thursday night. And the rest of the time *The Cunninghams* will be floaters, and sit wherever chance leads them.

Once a month it was Birthday Night in the dining room. All the birthday folk sat together at a special table, got complimentary champagne or wine. Then everybody sat down to a prime rib dinner, and birthday cake and ice cream. Another year crossed over to safety. So it was *Happy Birthday*, whether you gathered it up and tucked it in your pocket like a horse chestnut or rabbit's foot or lucky coin, or you ignored it altogether. A birthday was something. Just waking up alive was cause for communal celebration.

And watching over all was Donna, all five feet four inches of her, all 250 Irish pounds of her. She had a voice like a foghorn, a tattoo on her left shoulder. She went scuba diving in the Caribbean, took her grandchildren to Ireland, dreamed of snorkeling on the Great Barrier Reef. She loved every living soul in that place as they loved her. She kept them in line, prevented crowding, squabbles over who should sit where, made sure the music was loud enough to be heard but soft enough not to set off everybody's hearing aids.

Every second Tuesday of the month Donna ran the University House Food Service Discussion Group, or more accurately, the gripe session: the rolls are stale, beans overcooked, meat's tough, sausage too spicy, desserts too sweet. I hate fettuccine. Why can't we ever get fresh mango like I asked last time? My mother went to these meetings, if she could. In fact, at times she was the official note taker for the Residents' Association. She liked to say something nice to the chef, who stood at the podium beside Donna and took it all down. And because, in her words, it was always an "interesting experiment in human behavior." Though they were in the minority, these complainers were often the "characters" of University House, as my mother called them. People who could not wear their aging lightly or with grace, who felt the hovering presence of death more acutely than others, who held on to life's bitterness and regrets. People like my uncle.

But even these people had been places, done things: they were doctors, lawyers, college professors, nurses, a college president or two. There were no basket weaving or potholder classes, no stitch and snitch groups. There were political discussions, presentations, chamber music in the auditorium, classical music club, French club, Shakespeare club, poetry club, tai chi, yoga, stretch and flex, outings to museums, lectures, the opera, the theater, the ballet, if you could make it up the stairs of the bus. If you could sit that long without having to go to the bathroom or having your back give out.

All of this was more important to me than it was to my parents and my uncle. I wanted signs and symbols that they would remain as they had been, that they wouldn't become childlike, and spend their afternoons gluing macaroni and glitter to blue construction paper in an endless summer camp from which you never went home because you were already there.

So I went to sleep at night thinking of people at tai chi or the opera or the classical music club, even though my parents went to few of these things. See? You didn't just dump them anywhere. The lobby said that. The chandelier hanging from the high ceiling said that, and the presidential, navy blue carpet up the spiral staircase to the gallery, and the library with its Dale Chihuly glass and art exhibit, grand piano, brocade furniture, the *New York Times* on an oak spindle, porcelain chess set on the oak coffee table—all of it said you had not thrown them away, you had not forgotten them and laid them to rest. But my father didn't care a thing about all this; he was just glad they were all together in this safe place. And my mother. Something eased in her. She relaxed in some profound, though unstated way. Now there were others to catch them if they fell. I knew, though never said, that as much as this move was saving my father, it was saving her, and saving me too.

And so they settled into life at The House, and I think they were happy. Most of the residents were gracious, kind, intelligent, witty, cheerful, courageous in their determination to live with style and curiosity. But I wondered what it was like to live in a house where death was a fall, a sneeze, a heartbeat away. There was a dignity about these people, and an unspoken rule among them to assume the best face you could. No walking the halls in your bathrobe, no food stains down your front. There were appearances to keep. Yet eventually this one or that one began to slip. People fell down, were carried away, some out the side door forever, others out the front, to battle their way back from the hospital, rehab, to come home with twenty-four-hour care, before the move to assisted living, and only rarely to living completely on their own.

But it was sad to me that my parents as a couple did not make a single, abiding friendship. I did not know yet that this was dangerous business, and that for the most part people kept their attachments light. There were other couples my parents might have become friends with, one couple in particular, Bill and Ann Stylstra, who lived right across the hall from them. If my father had been his gregarious former self, and if my parents had been a twosome instead of a threesome, the couples might have struck up a gentle, easy friendship, become great friends, gone out to dinner together, to concerts, lectures. Bill was a retired college professor too. Yet it was really too late for all that, and as it turned out, too late for Bill too, because both men had winding down hearts.

But mostly I wished friends for my mother. She was the one who would need them. My mother was constantly attending to my father during those brief years at University House, and there was little occasion to make friends.

Just as I Am

They had always been religious. My mother and father and my uncle had all grown up in the Free Methodist Church, and all of them had gone to the Free Methodist Greenville College in Illinois. When my parents moved to Spokane they became Presbyterian, and in Michigan, my uncle became a nominal Episcopalian. So several months after my father's stroke, the three of them began to take up the threads of their lives as best they could, and resumed what now had become a virtually heroic effort to get to church on Sunday. It was a habit of a lifetime that even the treachery of those Spokane winters and my father's precarious footsteps could not prevent.

The smooth green hymnal with the gold lettering, held now in a shaky right hand, the response card in the little pocket on the back of each pew where you used to write your name and pass it to your neighbor to the left, the choir loft above the sanctuary and the brass organ pipes you could see if you turned your head, though it was better to just shut your eyes and let that sound float down upon you. The familiar, well-loved order of service—the introit, the call to worship, the scripture for the day, the sermon that applied the scripture to your everyday life even now, words just for you, as you sat there with what felt like half of you gone, then the final hymn, Presbyterian, steadfast and unadorned, and finally the recessional with the organ at full throttle, as you made your way out into the foyer, taking care to watch your step in all that rush of laughter and release. Then all the folks to greet you and ask after you, the coffee and cookies in the fellowship hall, which you now had to skip because of the stairs.

And so now with this move to Seattle, it was the first question to come up. Where would they go to church? And how would they get there? They wanted to go to the University Presbyterian Church a few miles away, a large church they had visited a few times before, and though they know no one, it would soon be like an old friend, or so they hoped. I'd called the church in advance and asked if there was a van or perhaps a group of volunteers who helped older people get to church. But I was told there was no such a thing.

That first Sunday they ordered a taxi and set off with my father in the front seat and my mother and uncle and my father's hand crutch in the back. These days my father was none too steady with just the hand crutch, though he fervently did not want to use his walker for church. But in the bustle of all the comings and goings in the church foyer, someone bumped his shoulder, and with only the hand crutch to steady himself, he almost toppled over. He felt himself going down and reached out and there was my mother, who grabbed his elbow and held on, but she could feel herself go forward too, and my uncle caught her arm and leaned back on his heels and somehow the three of them righted themselves. So after that first time my father came with his walker, though soon after he eased from the walker to the wheelchair without protest. None of them had wanted to call attention to their afflictions, but of course it could not be helped, as their collective infirmity called after them everywhere they went.

Of course there was a wheelchair ramp—how could there not be, with a church that size. And so for a little while, it was all right, though my uncle struggled to push my father up the ramp, as he was none too steady himself, and then after church he'd ease it back down the ramp to the waiting cab. Besides, with the wheelchair my father had a place to sit while they waited for the cab, my uncle dashing out every few minutes to see if the cab was there, furious, and in no time frantic.

So they negotiated the trip to and from church on their own in treacherous cab rides that exhausted them—the anxious wait for the cab, hoping it would not be too late—they needed to get there before the press of the crowd—but not too early so they wouldn't have to sit too long. Then at last the cab would come and my uncle would help my father edge his way into the front seat while the driver shoved the wheelchair into the trunk. Then after the service another wait, hoping the cab would come before my father slumped over in fatigue.

Then one Sunday, coming down the ramp after church, my uncle almost lost control of the wheelchair, staggering after it with his jerky, eighty-five-year-old steps and nothing to halt the gathering momentum of the wheelchair toward that busy street. *Help, help!* he'd wanted to call, but only my mother noticed my uncle's plunging gait as he tried to slow down the wheelchair, my father's eyes, wide and disbelieving, and that grimace my father always used to tease us with for real now. "*Henry!*" he cried out, "*Henry!*"

That was the day they gave up on University Presbyterian Church, the renowned church with the prestigious minister, the famous choir, the massive sanctuary. And the whole time no one ever came to visit them and welcome them into the fold, or ask how can we help. They were embraced by no one, nor welcomed or remembered. All those people rushing past in their Sunday best, and no one to ask after them or say their name. All dressed up, which was part of their ritual too, in their Sunday best, and no one to notice how fine they looked.

These images are as poignant to me now as they were then, and coming with only a little less guilt. I could have been that volunteer to get them to church. But some way I could not be the volunteer they never found. The reasons are tangled, and I'm not sure I understand them all myself. All I know is that my heart closed up against it. Even knowing what a great gift it would be to them, to my father especially, I could not do it. How my father would have loved it, having us all together. He could watch how intently we were listening to the sermon, how our heads bowed in prayer. He'd have checked to see that our eyes were closed. It seems like a simple thing to have done, looking back on it now. *Desideratum.* The heart's desire. I could not become their heart's desire.

Thinking of it now, it would have taken the entire morning just getting there and back, and then there would be an after-church Sunday brunch, somewhere crowded and familiar, then the usual errands for their groceries, drugstore needs. The day would go on and on. And how shamed I was when a friend offered to take them to church instead of me.

But University Presbyterian Church was just too big and too far away, they decided, too many people, and cars and little kids not looking their way. Maybe a smaller church would be best. Someone at The House had told them of a little neighborhood Presbyterian church a few blocks from their apartment, a little brick building whose stairs my father struggled to negotiate with only his hand crutch, as there was no handicapped ramp, and so no way to use a wheelchair or even a walker. And then one Sunday soon after, he fell trying to go up those stairs.

After that there was no more going to church on Sunday ever again, unless you counted the church services held in the nursing home where my father spent the last two months of his life. And so on Sunday mornings at ten, the three of them turned to *The Crystal Cathedral* or some such TV program for church. They sat in those three chairs curved around the television, bowed in prayer along with the people on television. It was a step up from the Holy Roller version of religious broadcasting, but to me it was still show business, and so it made me sad and a little angry to think of this poor substitute for what they had always loved so much. But the anger was only guilt turned inside out since I was really only angry at myself.

But the guilt of it lessened quickly as their needs became increasingly more complex and more urgent. And Sunday was already their day. My husband and I would do the weekly grocery shopping, run their drugstore errands, and then take them all out to dinner Sunday night. No need to add church to all that. No time anyway, with school the next day and all the class preparations and papers left undone. Thus I could remain the good daughter even so. But my reluctance to take them to church bothered me long after they had given it up, as it does to this day. I think the beginning of that resistance goes all the way back to my early childhood years growing up in that little college town in southern Illinois.

"Are you saved?" It was a question that had haunted my father all his life, as it had his father before him, as my grandfather's job as Free Methodist minister was "bringing in the sheaves." But this question took on a greater urgency in my father's last years, as one ailment begat another. He felt sure of his own salvation but worried over the rest of us. *Are you saved, Henry? All you whom I love, are you saved?* His greatest fear was that we would be torn from him at the Great Divide, never to see us again. After all, he'd grown up a preacher's kid and had given many sermons over the years himself as a lay preacher in churches with a pastor on leave or on vacation.

Ed and I did not go to church. Ed had served as altar boy until he grew too much, too fast, and kept passing out at the communion rail when he leaned over then straightened back up. When he was twelve he wanted to be a priest. Maybe every altar boy goes through this phase, which, happily for my sake, was a short one. Both of us had been forced by our parents to attend Sunday church, Mass, Bible School, Sunday School, midweek prayer group, choir, catechism classes, and both of us were ready to be done with all that.

But when our children came along, some song from the past rang in our ears. Abide with me. So Ed and I added his Catholicism to my Presbyterianism, and it came out Lutheran. A little more liturgy for me, a little more sermon for him. So we went to Lutheran classes and joined the Prince of Peace Lutheran Church, invited my parents for the weekend from Spokane to see the children baptized. They stood with us in front of the congregation and promised to help raise the children in the ways of the Lord. I remember looking over at my father and seeing the tears in his eyes. I imagined he was thinking of his own father then, and all the baptisms he had performed, and the comfort and safety of promises made and promises kept. Each child received a baptismal handkerchief, which had been used to wipe the holy water from their foreheads, which should have been kept but was lost in the flotsam of life. Chris was eight, Robb was six, and Courtney was almost two, which says we'd waited longer than we should have for safety's sake. Along with vitamins and seatbelts and nutritious food and looking both ways and holding hands when we crossed, baptism was a good thing. Better than a rabbit's foot or good luck charm or totem in your pocket. Holy water didn't wash away my children's sins for me. They were already perfect. Still, I thought of it as a cobalt blue shield, a ritual of protection against accident and disease and the cruelty of bullies and name-callers, and bad luck of every kind.

And as those years played out we tried mightily to take them to church. The children hated it. They thought the liturgist sounded like Kermit the Frog and had to stifle their laughter every time he began to sing. They drew, played tic-tac-toe while they waited for Kermit the Frog to sing again. Eventually, even the promise of Winchell's Donuts after church was not enough to keep us in the fold.

And so we quit the church. And that's where we were when my father began to feel the closing of his life and the pressure of saving us if he could, before he died. Our nonchurchgoing ways troubled him deeply, because my father's narrowing sense of the visible proof of salvation was church attendance. My father's belief was so absolute and anguished he couldn't bear the thought of anyone being outside the grace of God, and yet his belief told him that many were. And what if those he loved were outside the circle of salvation as well? Time was running out for my father to save us, and now he might lose us for good. We could be separated from him for all eternity.

"Are you leaving enough time for Jesus?" my father sometimes asked me, not as a reproach, but with an apprehension and a profound sadness. "Oh yes, of course I am," I'd say, glad he did not ask for specifics, glad we could move on for a while, until the doubts built themselves up again in the darker reaches of his mind. And then once again, the anguished look would come just before the drop in his voice asking for reassurance that all was spiritually well. Or with the kids. Sometimes when my parents came to Seattle for a visit, my father would knock on their bedroom door, and when they opened it and said, "Hi Grandpa," he'd ask, in the same kind and anguished manner, "Have you let Jesus into your heart?" And they would respectfully say, "Sure, Grandpa, sure." Their answer was always a gift of love he did not recognize.

Though he asked me these things from time to time, and more rarely the kids, he never questioned my husband, the former Catholic, who always remained something of a mystery to him. With Ed, he left such intrusions alone. Maybe he recognized that for Ed such a question would have no context. Catholicism was a foreign world to my father. He could see my husband's separateness, and respected it. But with us, he could never see where he left off and we began. Being an identical twin, how could it be otherwise? And so we bore his occasional, evangelical intrusions as best we could. It was all right. They were gentle, graceful questions that slipped in and out of my children's lives, though I think those things found their way into secret places in their minds and hearts after all, for my children all came to possess a spirituality they could not name. Still, the question had haunted me, also, because however being saved was supposed to feel, I was sure I had never felt it.

Neither had my uncle. I knew even as a child that there was something about my uncle, my glamorous, worldly uncle, that worried my father deeply. Maybe it was all his girlfriends. My parents joked about them, but there was something under the joking that was dark and fearful to my father, though it somewhat amused my mother.

As a child, I went to church with my parents every Sunday. I was this little soul whose heart had tried and tried to come to God, but who remained on the edge of uncertainty. I would try everything I could think of to be sure my uncle—whom I loved as much as I loved my parents—had been saved. I said prayers for him if not for myself. And so my father's fears had become my own. My uncle had felt a profound sense of unworthiness his whole life, which accounted for his efforts at self-importance that were so often a trial to us. Later, I thought of my uncle whenever I heard the words I'd borrowed from my husband's Catholicism: *I am not worthy that you should come under my roof. Say but the word and my soul shall be healed.*

But as it happened, a few years before he died, my uncle announced that after years of trying, he had been saved at last. There was no fanfare or weeping at the altar, just a quiet turning of the heart he'd gently reported to my parents one morning at breakfast.

Are you saved? That question touched a nerve I was always surprised to find still there. When my father entered his revivalist mode, I always wanted to run from the room. Post-traumatic church disorder, I'd always called it. I believed in certain things, but they remained private, and could not be brought out for accounting. I was not faithless entirely. But I had never had the sine qua non for salvation—the mountaintop experience, as it was called in my father's Southern, evangelical world, where you went up the mountain one person and came down another.

It was the summer I was nine and we still lived in Greenville, Illinois, that little college town just across the Mississippi River from St. Louis, where my parents both taught. It was called the "Children's Revival." It was a special service to save the children, held every summer in the church sanctuary. But why were children in need of saving? What was there in a child that needs to be saved? Everything, if you believe in the age of knowing, which said that after you turned twelve you were responsible for everything you did and could be damned to hell for things you didn't even know you'd done. My father assured me during my childhood night terrors that I was years away from the age of knowing, and so I was safe in the arms of God just for being who I already was. But I could count, and knew that eventually I would turn a corner and there I would be, face to face with eternity.

We were all gathered in the main sanctuary of the church, having come up from our basement classrooms where we were in the middle of Vacation Bible School. The windows were open and a soft afternoon breeze fluttered through the sanctuary. I was sitting about halfway back with my friend Janie Hasenmeyer. We were listening to the man on the stage, the revivalist, who was telling us about our need to repent for our sins and let Jesus into our hearts.

But I had stopped listening to the words because I was caught up in the sound of his voice, the way it went up and down in that rhythmic crooning way, like a love song sung just for you. The organist was playing "Softly and tenderly Jesus is calling, calling for you and for me," while the ladies' choir hummed along in the background. Kids here and there were beginning to cry. I was holding on tightly to myself against that tug and pull I felt in my heart, this calling up. I could hardly swallow. My eyes ached. Jesus was calling for *me*. There was a sweet and terrible power in these words that was different from "Onward Christian Soldiers," which we sang at the beginning of every Vacation Bible School day.

Then the revivalist announced the *altar call*. "Those among you who wish to be saved by the Blood of the Lamb, come forward *now*. Walk down that aisle and come to the altar, to kneel before *Jesus* and confess your sins." His voice had changed. Now it was urgent, fierce, commanding. I was carried along by that rhythm, more insistent now, every third or fourth syllable ringing like a brass note I could feel spinning darkly inside my head. That rhythm took over my mind and erased all thought and will. Then the choir began the endless choruses of "Just as I Am." It didn't ask us to be soldiers. It asked for something deeper. It was hypnotic. It was irresistible, like grace itself. It was simple yet grown up, and carried a kind of gentle eroticism I would only identify years later. And once you'd heard it, that song would speak your name forever, gather your breath in such tender hands, and wrap you in such sweetness and longing you were not the singer any longer, but the song.

Just as I am
without one plea
but that thy blood was shed for me.
Blessed Jesus, I come, I come.

His eyes were soft and bright and full of tears, the sweat rolling down his dark, dark face. How he wanted us to be saved. How he was loving us into it. The sound of that voice going up and down to the rhythm of those wavery female voices matching his pulled us against our willing toward that altar and the confessions that would save our souls. Suddenly, I was kneeling at the altar. I had no idea how I'd gotten there. No memory of walking down the center aisle of the church to that beckoning, waiting altar, that half circle of mahogany that rimmed the stage. No memory of finally getting up my courage and rising from my seat. I was just sitting in the pew, trying to hold the tears back, and then the next minute I was kneeling at the altar crying my heart out. I had not decided to do this; I had just done it.

I had never cried in public before that I could remember. I had seen this often enough, and was mostly fascinated and appalled by this bringing what was inside to the outside, this communal revelation of rapture and pain. What had happened to me? Had I let Jesus into my heart? How did I get there without even knowing it? I was suddenly kneeling at the altar like all the other kids, crying for no reason I could name. Even Jimmy Horton, the terror of the fourth grade, was at the altar sobbing his heart out. Now I was saved. I was at that altar. I had come.

"Have you been saved before?" the volunteer said to me, as she knelt beside me and touched my neck. I shivered. Her hand was cold. *Before*? Was I saved *before*? I was shocked. I didn't know. Didn't this only happen once in your whole life?

"Have you been saved before?" she said again.

"I don't know. I don't think so. Maybe."

Saul into Paul. A blinding light on the road to Damascus. A new sense of things. I'd heard enough sermons by then to know I had not changed from one thing into another. Born again? I was not born again. I felt exactly as I had always been. There had been no right angles in my life, no stark turns. If I had been an alcoholic, or a drug addict, or a murderer, maybe then I would notice the change. But my life was too ordinary for anything as dramatic as that. If I had been born again, I did not know it. I hated things that changed. Being born again, though it meant my salvation, terrified me almost as much as the thought of going to hell. What would it matter where I went if I didn't know who I was? What would it matter where I went if I stopped being me?

Then the volunteer asked me to confess my sins. I tried hard to think of things that would damn me to hell in another three years when I turned twelve but could only think of one. "I play dress-up," I said. And thinking this needed more weight, more sinfulness, I explained about the college girls. At that time I lived in the women's dorm. My mother was dean of women then, and we had a little apartment at the end of the hall, and my room was a dorm room. My parents had made it into a child's bedroom, like any other. Except it had its own vanity and sink. I remember washing my socks in that sink when I walked home in the rain without my shoes because they were new and I didn't want to get them wet and then I lied about it. Maybe that was the sin.

I was a little mascot, a little pet with the girls, and they would give me their skirts and sweaters and shoes and nightgowns for playing dress-up, when they were packing up for the summer. They would throw the rest in the dumpsters just outside the back of the dorm. I would climb out the window at the end of the hall and down the fire escape to the back lot where the throwaway clothes were. Janie and I would pile up the clothes until we could hardly carry the load home. Nothing to go to hell for, but it came tumbling out on a virtual flood of tears as if it were the biggest sin on earth. It was the sin of worldliness, the sin of adornment. I cried all the way to Janie's house, where we stood in her backyard and cried some more. I remembered the chicken her father had beheaded that had come running right toward me earlier that summer, blood spurting out of its severed neck. We were standing by the tree stump where he had done it, and somehow the memory of that chicken rushing toward me came back to me and was connected to the words of that song that were now no longer plaintive but terrible in the shedding of blood.

Just as I am without one plea
But that thy blood was shed for me.

The theology always seemed wrong to me. The denial of the things of this world always struck me as both too easy and too hard. I'd always understood the allure of worldliness. I'd wanted to join a circus, wear pink tights and sequins and makeup, and fly through the air. I loved lipstick and nail polish and jewelry of any kind. All things considered worldly and sinful in that time and place. I loved it that my mother had a secret tube of red lipstick tucked away in her purse for when we went to St. Louis. She could never wear it in Greenville, though she let me try it on when I played dress-up. Of course when we moved to Spokane and became Presbyterian, she could wear all the makeup she wanted. But that tube of lipstick for St. Louis trips was part of her rebelliousness that I loved. Yet if worldliness was indeed a sin, it must have been the same sin that kept my uncle from being saved also, with his new cars and beautiful clothes, his theater tickets and his girlfriends. I wanted that worldliness too, but only had visions of it in the throwaway pile of clothes behind the girls' dorm.

I often wondered what those girls did, how their lives differed from mine, what they talked about behind their closed doors. I also wondered what my mother's work with them was. What was a dean of women anyway? I had no idea. Girls came and went into her office, sometimes closing the door. My father had a little adjoining office where he was often at work writing his doctoral dissertation, a fan blowing on his bare feet. He'd clap his hands above his head to work through writer's block, though he would never have used that term. Through the door of that little adjoining office, I could sometimes hear crying and my mother's low, cool voice that made it stop. I remembered my mother's description of the pranks she pulled in her own college days: Vaseline on toilet seats and door handles, short-sheeting beds, hidden alarms set to go off at four in the morning—and the trick she and her roommate played on the housemother of their dorm, an elderly retired missionary, one winter weekend when she was gone. On Friday night they filled her bathtub with packets of Jell-O, turned on the hot water, then opened her bathroom window to the frigid winter air. On Sunday night when she returned, there it was: a bathtub full of Jell-O. I wondered if that's what those girls had done. But somehow I knew their transgressions or sorrows were far beyond my imagining.

Yet if this was the age of knowing I had so feared, I knew I wanted it anyway. I would risk damnation for this kind of knowing. I could always repent later. It was all part of a mysterious world I had only hints of but whose secrets were literally living next door. I remember how we were awakened one night by a girl who'd discovered a tick on her belly after a campus hike and how I overheard the conjecture between my parents about how that tick had gotten there. Even then I wondered how a tick could have gotten underneath her shirt and pants. I would not understand until years later the connection between eroticism and spirituality, in rapture of any kind, and the way my mind had linked them both so early on to sin.

• • •

In his last years my father had ordered strange and startling books. Was this part of the brain damage no test could find? *How to Save Your Family from Satan* and books on demons and angels and other such things lay on the bookstand by his bed, which alarmed my children on his account as well as their own, but it made me mostly sad. Where was my intellectual father, my NYU PhD father now? He knew time was running out. We didn't understand why he needed those books that shocked and offended us. He was nearing the thin place and we could not read the translation.

But in things of the spirit, all of us led thoughtful lives where art and the expression of art became part of our spiritual life, a life that he could not understand and that could not be shared with him. *Have you let Jesus into your heart?* I suppose looking back on it, there was something extraordinary in that altar call after all, a moment of purity in all that dross. Or maybe I was only remembering it thus as a way to reclaim the part of my father that now seemed so lost to me.

Did he, at the very end, think he was going to a place that would separate him from us for all eternity? When speech left him and he could no longer talk about God or anything else or ask us the questions that had lain so heavily on his heart all those years—was he finally at peace? Or did he believe he would lose us? That we would lose him? Maybe that was the reason he had so much trouble, in the end, letting us go.

Loving Uncle Henry

My parents looked forward to our Sunday dinners all week, though for us they were often tricky and difficult times. We might have looked forward to them in the same way, if we had truly known how little time we had left. You think you can imagine that kind of final absence, but you can't. With everybody tucked safely inside the present moment, that ultimate silence is only theoretical. How can it be otherwise? Deep within the logical mind, you're safe from your anguished heart.

So once in a while, when things had gone reasonably well, and no one had choked or insulted the waiter or fallen down, and we were all quiet, just watching the water, or finishing up the meal, I would look at my father as he watched out the window, where we sat at Anthony's, my father's favorite restaurant, overlooking Puget Sound. I wanted that moment to go on forever—the sun slipping down behind the Olympic Mountains in the distance, backlighting the clouds with pink and gold, and sailboats and motor boats making their way quickly homeward toward the canal in the last of the light, and a little later the tugboats and ferries, and an occasional cruise ship lit up against the night, floating by in the distance, or pulling across the water toward the open sea. All safe, all safe. For now, all safe.

I could leave it like this, and that would be the end of it. Because what followed, if seen from a great and forgiving distance, is the slow, tender fade of those last months, when the twins lived with my mother in that two-bedroom apartment at University House. Yet there must be some insight to come out of the raw details of those months, the ones we would turn from if we could. My mother reminds me of my duty to tell the whole story. She wants to understand the arc of their lives, how things came together and then came apart. And so do I.

But it is not easy going. It was strange how much my uncle's presence in our lives changed things, yet how much love there was even so. My uncle was so difficult those last years, and my parents gave up so much to have him there. It had seemed so anguished at the time, but in fact it has left no bitterness. My mother wants to understand if there was something given back, after so much was given up. She wants to make peace with all that might have been and was not—the trips my parents could have taken, the concerts, operas, theater they would have had together, how they loved the pleasure of the other's company, how, for the last twenty years, my uncle came along everywhere they went, how they couldn't bear to leave him behind.

I think of how I longed to have my parents to myself once in a while those last years, and how relieved I often was when my uncle declined the dinner out to stay behind. He was such a trial, and there were so many ways now for things to go wrong. Yet I have never been able to explain to others how I loved him, or explain why it was my parents had willed me to him. If something had happened to them, I would go to him. My bachelor Uncle Henry, who had many girlfriends but no wife, many students who loved him, but no child. Except for me. He rounded out our little family of three, made it the four of us on every vacation or holiday we ever had. He was my almost father. He looked like my father, talked like my father, laughed like my father, even smelled like my father. And that's exactly how I loved him.

When I was very little I thought all fathers came in pairs. A dashing father with a dashing identical twin brother. One light, one dark; one happy, one sad. My father was full of faith and light; my uncle full of shadows and doubt. My uncle's legacy from the South was a subtle racism he tried to overcome but could not. My father had no such struggles. My uncle had always felt that their parents preferred my father. And maybe they did. My father was joyful in ways my uncle never was.

But my uncle did not go gently into the night of old age. He railed at the dark, and it made him formidable to everyone who didn't know him. He could not accommodate change. "But, Uncle Henry, if you want to get hold of us just leave a message."

"But why would I leave you a message if you aren't home?" Behind his back my children and I called him "the evil twin." How that appellation became a term of endearment I cannot explain. But it was.

Because of him, those family dinners out were often fraught with complications I could not have faced in an unmedicated state. I would have ordered an immediate glass of wine, if I had not been allergic to alcohol. So I depended on that prophylactic little yellow pill—*for anxiety, take as needed.* Then I could coast through dinners serene as could be. It even got me through the minor choking episodes both my father and uncle regularly had at meals, as well as my uncle's insulin moments. And by now, both my uncle and my father were insulin-dependent diabetics—my father first, in his early sixties, which we all blamed on his sugar-loving ways. How we loved to kid him then, as we watched him put spoonful after spoonful of sugar in his coffee, or drink Eagle Brand condensed milk straight from the can, having no idea what he was doing to himself because of it. When he was finally banned from sugar forever, he used to say that sometimes walking through a store he'd wanted to reach into the candy bins and grab a handful. No more oatmeal cookies with raisins, no strawberry shortcake or apple pie or homemade ice cream with chocolate sauce. My uncle had no such sweet tooth, and so, though doctors told him for years that if his brother had diabetes he had to have it too, it did not make itself known until ten years after my father's diagnosis. Now they were identical twins in this too.

And thus the problem of when and where to take the before-dinner insulin injection, to be administered half an hour to forty-five minutes before a meal, but not much longer, or the risk was low blood sugar. And it was tricky, because you could never tell for certain when you were going to be putting that first bite of food in your mouth. My father had always excused himself and gone into the bathroom to take his insulin, as did my uncle. After the stroke, my mother had worked out a discreet way to give my father his before-dinner insulin injection at the table so smooth and quick you had to be watching for it to see that needle at all.

My uncle was another matter. He used that moment as a weapon to rage against the night. He would inject himself in plain view at the table in the middle of the restaurant, no matter how much we protested. I have always been needle phobic, and so I came to dread this moment, as my uncle was anything but discreet.

"But, Uncle Henry," I said, "couldn't you do this right before we leave for the restaurant? It's only a fifteen-minute ride."

"But what if we got in a car accident?"

"We won't get in an accident. We'll be careful."

"Grace gives it to Homer at the table."

"But he's had a stroke. Before his stroke he did it in the bathroom. Couldn't you do it in the bathroom like you used to?"

He remembered the time someone yelled at my father in the bathroom and accused him of shooting up drugs, and how angry and embarrassed he had been.

So no, Uncle Henry would not take his insulin injection at the apartment or in the restaurant men's room. He would take it at the table, like my father. After we had been seated and ordered our food, he would retrieve his insulin syringe and needle out of his coat pocket and roll up his shirt and inject himself in the white, fatty part of his abdomen. I could not watch. I'd scan the restaurant to see who might be looking, and thankfully nobody ever was. But I had never seen anyone do this, not before, not since.

But now and then it went something like this: just as my uncle was poised to inject, the server would arrive at the table with the salad course. He'd set the tray down and turn to serve the first salad.

"Do you want some of my *insulin*?" my uncle would say, waving the needle in the air. The server would turn pale and back away, the plate of salad still in his hands. Rarely was there a comeback for such a line. Then someone with more experience would arrive and serve the salads. By then the syringe and needle were safely back in my uncle's coat pocket and his shirt was more or less tucked back in.

It's strange now, how writing this I feel nothing but tenderness for him. I cannot bring into view the frustration and anger I had at the time. Of course, it was all part of that slowing down, of that inevitable letting go of earthly matters, like spotless clothes, decorum, and kindness to strangers.

So it was complicated, and though that needle at the dinner table distressed me, he was old now, and I told myself he couldn't help it, whether or not it was true. But I loved him so much I could eventually forgive him anything. He was my beloved uncle. When I had turned my face away and was counting to twenty, I tried to remember how much I had loved him when I was a little girl. I would bring up an image or two, and then it was all right. How we would go to meet his train at night come down from Michigan to Illinois for Christmas, and I would sit on my knees in the backseat of the car, so excited my stomach hurt, counting the mile markers until we arrived at the train station. And I would run to meet him and he'd gather me up and carry me back to the car. "I have a present for you," he'd say. "It's a *garment*."

"Oh, what is it? What is a *garment*?" I'd shout. Of course I knew what it was. But it was our little script. It was a white dress with frills and lace. Or a pink and white-striped sundress, which I wore to Bible School because my very own Uncle

Henry was coming from Michigan to pick me up, only the girl next to me was coughing so hard I thought she would throw up all over it before my uncle could see how pretty I looked in that dress he'd sent me in the mail.

Or a plaid wool Easter cape and matching cap, like nothing any of my friends ever had. There is a picture of me wearing that cape and little cap in a silver frame on my uncle's desk. In the picture I'm standing on a ledge, holding an Easter lily, smiling into the face of the one who is smiling at me, and it's either my uncle or my father sitting on the ledge with his arm around my waist. My uncle always claimed he was the one in the picture, since he was the one who had given me the cape and little cap. My mother and father went along with him, but it came up in argument now and then anyway.

"Oh, it doesn't matter which one of us it is, Henry," my father would finally say, wanting to end the disagreement between them.

"*Yes*, it does. *I'm* the one in the photograph."

I knew exactly who it was, but kept it to myself. Of course it was my father. Their likenesses only went so far. They weren't interchangeable to me. They weren't a doubling either. If you are lucky enough to be so loved, your face is like no other. Even as a little girl, I knew there really was no such thing as identical twins.

But the fact that they were so alike helps explain in part how nothing my uncle ever did, no matter how egregious, could diminish how much I loved him. He was as precious to me now as he was when I was that little girl in the photograph with my father, in the Easter cape he'd bought for me.

My uncle came with us every summer on all our long road trips across the country from Illinois to Washington to see my maternal grandparents. We played Brain Surgery most of the way. I'd use his comb and pen to operate, and his handkerchief and spare Kleenex to bandage him up, which mainly meant me laying the handkerchief across his face so he could sleep it off. On those long trips, with my mother and father in the front seat and my uncle and I in the backseat, he was my playmate, my companion, the siblings I did not have. I was never lonely on those long trips, and when Brain Surgery ended because his hair began to thin, we played Jukebox. I'd put a nickel in his shirt pocket and he was supposed to sing whatever I wanted him to, but, unlike my father with his beautiful tenor voice, my uncle couldn't carry a tune and knew hardly any songs. So all that jukebox would play was "The Old Gray Mare" and "All I want for Christmas Is My Two Front Teeth." I would scream with feigned anger and delight because when we invented that game I had no front teeth.

In our family the stories about my uncle are legendary, and my children loved hearing about Uncle Henry in the past, but they also collected their own stories about him to be brought out whenever they wanted to be the hit of the party with their friends, or to remind them that even this embarrassment or that would make a great story in the end. To my parents he was often like a misbehaving child, but a child they loved unconditionally nonetheless. The story of my uncle is the story of my parents too, and their abiding love for him.

For many years, in addition to teaching history and being a school administrator, my uncle was a championship debate coach. Maybe this explains why in old age debate became his métier, with its defense, attack, counterattack. He loved to start a controversy or an argument whenever he could. It was his odd way of relating to us, I guess, though no one really understood it or knew where it came from, this combative way of expressing affection—some legacy from that twinned childhood maybe or those undemonstrative parents who chose one twin over the other.

It usually began with a seemingly innocent question, and always in restaurants. "Robb," he'd say to my artist son, "what do you think of that painting over there?" He's pointing to the Jackson Pollock–style painting against the wall on the other side of the restaurant. "I think that's junk."

There is no right answer and my son knows it. Robb is not particularly fond of the painting either, but he doesn't want to agree with his uncle on that. My uncle doesn't get a reaction, so he pushes on. "What do you think of pornography in art?" He's warming up to it, becoming more animated all the time.

Robb makes some defense of artistic freedom in all things. He can't help himself now, and my uncle's counting on this. Then my uncle references Serrano's *Piss Christ*. "So what do you think of *that*?"

But my son isn't going to bite. He knows what's coming and he's not going there. "I'm not going to get in an argument with you, Uncle Henry," he says with as much control as he can muster.

"Well, what about pictures of people having *sex with animals*." My uncle's voice rises on the last phrase just as the server arrives with the food. The waiter turns on his heels and goes right back to the kitchen, too stunned to notice he is still carrying the tray of food. My daughter bolts from the table in tears and rushes to the bathroom. She's fifteen, and since she's out with her family she wants to be invisible anyway. She's already embarrassed just by being here.

Then it's three years later and she's home from college for the weekend. These days she can sit through the meal no matter what topic comes up.

So my uncle asks, "What percentage of girls at your college have babies in the bathroom and stuff them in the trash can?"

My daughter laughs in disbelief. "Uncle Henry!" she says. She's all grown up now and won't be undone.

"Oh, I'll bet it's more than you think." He's either read some tragic piece in the paper or heard a segment on the news. She manages to hold on to her new grown-up sophistication and only rolls her eyes. Then she says more softly than he deserves, "Uncle Henry, that's not nice."

The children had a contest for years over who had the most outrageous Uncle Henry story, until my daughter finally won this contest and it was retired for good. The contest was a way for the children to make our meals out with him bearable, to hold their embarrassment in check, and to stop it from diminishing their love. And so we learned to see a good story in the making even as we were living it. They were stories that could save our love from the erosion that his old age exacted upon him and upon us. What is a story anyway, but a casting of raw, bitter facts into arcs of light?

My daughter calls because she's sure she has the winning Uncle Henry tale. She's out of college now, on her own. She and her boyfriend have taken the three-some to my parents' favorite little Mexican restaurant—favorite, meaning the one place they can get to on their own, if my father rides his motorized cart, my uncle uses his cane, and my mother watches her step. It's about two blocks up from University House. They arrive every Saturday at noon, so the staff at the restaurant have come to expect them, and have prepared a table just for them, with extra little bowls of salsa for my father, and extra napkins. It is kind and lovely, but my parents are concentrating so hard on just making it up those two blocks with no one tipping over that the staff's efforts go unnoticed. My father motors in the door and around the bend and up to their appointed table—no need to be seated for these regulars.

"You won't believe it, Annis P," my daughter says over the phone. It's what she calls me now. "Nobody will ever top this one." She's just come from lunch with the threesome at Beso del Sol. She has already converted trauma, humiliation, and shame, into laughter. She's tucked it away safely now where it can do no harm. Over time her storytelling will turn it into myth that will heal her. And it will heal me, so that I can go on to tell it now.

My father and mother order the Tombstone Burrito, which they'll share. My uncle orders his usual *hamburger*, plain. He hates this restaurant. He hates Mexican food. He hates all ethnic food in fact, all food he does not understand. It's more than this, though. He's afraid of otherness, of everything and everyone not like him, which these days is practically everybody. It's that conflicted racism he's struggled with his whole life. And the coffee's cold. Or it is now. He totters across the restaurant waving his cup. He puts his finger in it and announces to the whole restaurant, "This coffee is utterly *cold.*"

The staff rushes to replace it with a new cup of hot coffee, which he promptly cools down with a piece of ice from his water glass, because now, of course, it's too hot. But soon they're all busy with their lunch, their huge Mexican lunch, except for the hamburger. My father has consumed, by himself, his three little bowls of salsa and wants to order more. My mother has tucked under his chin a big cloth napkin she brings for just this occasion. It was a Christmas gift from my daughter, who has been to the Mexican lunch a time or two in the past and knows what my father's shaky hand does with those spoonfuls of salsa.

Maybe it's all the spices in the salsa or maybe it's just another lingering effect of the stroke, but my father precipitously, suddenly, turns to my mother and announces, "Grace. I have to go to the bathroom." She knows what he means. This isn't a little sweet pee. He's got Depends for that. This is the big one. My mother registers nothing. It's not like this hasn't happened before. But she's tired, and this will require a lot of work and she's really enjoying her burrito, extra beans no rice. "Lorin," she says to my daughter's boyfriend, "can you help him?"

"Sure," he says. Whatever he is to do he will do gladly, though he really has no idea what that is.

Because it happens now and then, we think this urgency has something to do with lack of sensation, or synapses in the brain, or maybe just anybody getting old. How it all comes down to this—a rising of the spirit that comes from the betrayals of the body, so that shame can fall away.

(I know I shouldn't make comparisons with the dog, but I can't help it. Alex, our beloved family dog, whose droppings soil the hall downstairs in the morning, is losing feeling in her hind end too. Often I think she doesn't even know it's happening. Or maybe her back hurts too much to go up the stairs to get outside through the dog door. At first she just turned her head and wouldn't look at us, shamed as she was. Now she just looks at us with surprise. *Now how did that happen? I wonder who did that?* We aren't angry at her, just weary of it all and a little sad. "It's okay," we tell her. After you are gone, after we lose you for good, we'll just rip up the carpet and start over, if we have to.)

Now my father is backing up his scooter and eventually manages to turn it around, though all this takes way too much time. But then he gets it pointed forward toward the bathroom, past rows of tables on both sides of the aisle. He's single-minded now, in a race against time. He's hunched over the handlebars like he's in a bumper car race in a cartoon. But he's angled slightly off-center and catches the corner of the first table and pulls the tablecloth off as he goes on by. Glasses and silverware go flying. He presses on. All he can think of is getting there in time. And so he barrels forward, crashing into table after table, leaving devastation in his wake. He's only concentrating on the goal line, or maybe he panics and can only remember how to go forward, can only think of that one urgent, overwhelming thing—to avoid shame. He has wiped out the whole upper level of the restaurant. My mother has gotten up to follow. It's too late for anything now, but there she goes. The staff is already on the scene, picking things up. "I'm sorry," my mother says, and hurries on. She'll head on into the men's room. She's been there too many times before. Lorin turns around to look at us as wide-eyed as a person can be, before he disappears behind her into the bathroom too.

My daughter and uncle are the only ones left at the table now. He strikes up a conversation. How he has gotten from the catastrophe that has just happened to this thought I cannot imagine. "So. Tell me, Courtney, who am I to you? I mean who do you think of me as?" That's easy. She loves him. Despite everything. Despite the *evil twin* nomenclature.

"Oh," she says instantly, "I've always thought of you as another grandfather." It's a lovely thing to say and comes as close to describing his special status as she can think of, since there is no name for who he is to my children or to me. My uncle should turn to her and say, "Why thank you, Courtney. That's wonderful."

But he doesn't. The silence hangs between them. She's waiting for the loving thing he's going to say back. She turns to see when everybody's coming back, not sure how long she can keep this up.

Just then the server comes to refill my uncle's coffee, keep this man's coffee *hot*, keep this man in his seat. And just then my uncle turns to her and says, "But then that would mean I'd have to have had *sex* with your grandmother."

The server hasn't heard a word. No sirree. Not a word. He's gone now, with the coffee pot and the empty bowls of salsa. He'll return to replenish the chips. Nothing can surprise him now.

But I wonder: what filter has worn so thin that it catches none of this before it goes out into the world? Oh, what does it mean? My uncle has never said anything like this before. He has never been anything but decorous and considerate with my mother. I wonder if this is a sign of an approaching dementia, some dark turn in personality that would take him beyond our ability to love him.

Yet every Saturday, the table set for them, the extra bowls of salsa for my father, the extra napkins, the familiar greeting, the genuine hello. No rolling of eyes. No audible sighs. No banishment. You can't come here anymore. After all, my uncle had already been evicted from the beauty salon at The House for some final, insufferable comment the hairdresser could not abide.

So there it is. All those things better left unsaid, doors to rooms better left unopened. But the story of my uncle is also the story of my parents and their absolute love for him, the way they took him in, and endured a hundred such offenses. And what did my parents sacrifice besides a little pride now and then in certain public places?

My husband and I have just come back from a little weekend getaway to Leavenworth, a kitschy, faux Bavarian town just over the mountains from Seattle. I call my mother the minute we return, just to be sure everything's all right.

"I have such fond memories of Leavenworth," my mother tells me.

"I know," I say.

"Do you know why we loved to go to Leavenworth? Because it's the one place your uncle didn't like," she says. "He wanted to come along everywhere else."

I am quiet, then change the subject slightly because I know what she's thinking. She's thinking about all the things lost between them, because of him. "Didn't Dad like to golf in Leavenworth?" I say stupidly. I know it's one of the great losses of her life, the times that might have been and were not, and right then I can't bear to hear her speak of it, not that she would.

"But you and Dad have a right to go off by yourselves," I used to argue back then, when this was still possible. "He's got to understand that." Did I know then how time was running out for them? I don't believe I did, even though my pleas were passionate. But it's my mother who says, "But he's so lonely. He doesn't have anyone but us." And so as much as they wanted to be by themselves they could not leave him behind. That pull and tug of one twin for the other may be incomprehensible to those outside the force field of twins, but my mother was wrapped in it, also, because of the way she loved my father.

The year or so before my father's stroke, my mother suffered a period of deep depression. "You seem sad all the time," I said. "What's making you so sad?" All she could say was that she was sorry she and my father hadn't been able to travel as much as they wanted. It was so slight, the way she said it, but I knew the depth of the loss she was mourning. In her understated way, there it was, their rich and abiding married life lived for years now on a narrower plane, in the unrecoverable loss of those years they might have had alone together.

The best trip of their retirement years did not include my uncle. It seems hard to believe this now, though my mother has the scrapbook to prove it. Ten years before my father's stroke, someone known only as "The Mystery Man" had given my parents an all-expenses-paid trip to anywhere in the world. Apparently he was a former Whitworth College student, whom my father had helped along the way. They never learned the identity of this man who paid for everything—a trip that started in England and ended in Italy three weeks later, with spending money for everything in between. Every so often when my mother is lonely she gets out the picture album she made of that trip and traces all the places they saw, places they stayed, meals they had. She'd written it all down day by day for safekeeping. That trip was the miracle of their retirement lives. Nothing would ever be that good again.

In these last years, the quieter my father became, the more animated became my uncle, removing forever the veil of that shifting yin and yang of twinhood. For even in their differences, they were in some essential way two halves of a whole. In this story my father and his quieter presence is eclipsed, and I struggle to bring him to life as he really was, and not as this catastrophe had made him.

Something is happening here. The spirit rises at times like these, the most egregious of times, when the mind becomes lost in the crises of the body. It rises and begins its separation from the betrayals of the body, on its way to someplace else. Given slightly different circumstances, we are all compelled by such betrayals. It is our imperious, extravagant pride that matters utterly for most of our lives—and matters so little at the end.

But we hold on to that sense of decorum for as long as we can, and criticize its loss in others, because that is what we fear most devoutly in ourselves—the missed step, the crumbs down the front of the blouse, the stains on the tie, the unbrushed hair, the button missed, the zipper undone, the dentures soaking in a glass on the sink, the wig placed decorously on its perfect, Styrofoam head, until we pass into the age of my uncle, where shame has been let go, not so much from neglect as from defiance and despair.

And so eventually there comes the inevitable slip and the whispered words of recognition: He's slipping. She's really slipping. Slipping on a banana peel, slipping in the bathtub, slipping through the catches of the mind, slipping through your fingers, your outstretched hands. But maybe it's not slipping so much, which has its own pejorative quality, as a shifting, a movement that carries no judgment and brings lessons of its own. The shadow that brushes across the face, the dark, widening eyes—a letting go of earthly things, the adornments of the body.

That's what these difficult years with my uncle have taught me. My parents could teach me no such lesson. They were always lovely and kind. Loving them back was no test of love. Loving my uncle was.

There is a set of blocks on the end table in back of the brocade couch in the foyer of the dining room at University House. You turn the blocks this way or that and create your own message. But it's a provocative mix. Turn the block one way and you get *G-o-d*, another *n-a-k-e-d*, another *s-e-x*, and yet another, *w-i-l-d w-o-m-e-n*. Ed and I and the kids always tried to come up with the most outrageous combination of words possible. We'd write some sentence with the words *wild women*, *sex*, and *love*, with the wish that everybody at one time or another before they checked out for good would have at least one of these, if not all three.

There are stories, of course, there always are, and occasionally a report in some magazine about what goes on behind closed doors in retirement communities. More power to them, my parents always said. The women here seemed to be forgiving of most things. A few had lowered their standards to meet what was at hand. And many women passed the new guy, whoever he was, without a second look. No thanks. No more taking care of old men. I'm done with all that.

My uncle had long given up wild women and sex. But it was a distant hope, and a little joke among us behind his back, that my uncle would find some age-appropriate woman who would see beyond the food stains on his sweater, his run-down shoes, his ungroomed hair, and see instead the man in the three-piece pinstriped suit with the handkerchief in his front pocket, the polished wingtips, the theater tickets in his pocket, see the man who was always teacher of the year wherever he went.

Once my uncle had loved a woman deeply and had asked her to marry him. But she rejected him and broke his wild and unguarded heart. He went to a dark place then and sought out a psychiatrist, who told him that his despair came from his mother, that she had never loved him. And so loving him or not, Alfreda shadowed the reach of his whole life. I will never marry, my uncle had said long ago. And he never did. It was a pronouncement just like Alfreda's, when she promised she would never smile again.

But my uncle had known Wild Women. It was one of the reasons all those years he could not be saved, because being saved would mean giving up sex with his girlfriends, and he could not do that. Imagine going through life believing it was either sex or salvation. But after the prostate surgery in his early seventies and the incontinence that followed, it all came to a sad and quiet end. And then saving grace at last. But all those years when he was never loved and never saved he was a throwaway person to himself, if not to others.

Early on I knew that sin and salvation were somehow bound up with sex, and my experience of the altar call only proved it. I remember writing a short story my sophomore year in high school, which I never showed anyone, called "My Uncle on Saturday Night," in which I imagined his wild and exotic sex life. But it was really more a coming-of-age story, about my own growing awareness of the complexities of sex, than a story about my uncle, though I didn't know it at the time. It was the same year I'd spent reading every Ian Fleming James Bond book there ever was. So much a mystery. I could barely imagine most of what I read, though I felt the pull of it as well as the fear.

It was not a secret during my adolescence that my uncle had lots of girl-friends. And why not? He was a bachelor, after all. I didn't realize for a long time, though, that for many of his girlfriends an exchange of money was required. Nor did I know how that might change the way men and women were together, or what my uncle paid those women to do. My uncle supposedly had kept a list of all the women he had slept with over the years. I wondered about the purpose of such a list. Maybe it was proof that he was loved in some way, that he was worthy of love of some kind. He'd told my father it was well over a hundred.

My mother is ill. She's known since the start that I'm writing a memoir of the twins and in some way her illness has loosened a fragment from her memory, and she offers it up with no segue whatsoever. "When you write about Henry, you should put this in." I wonder at first if the illness has let things out she'd otherwise have kept in, but somehow I don't think so. She too seeks understanding. And what she tells me is so rich, explains both so much and so little, I know it is a gift and a curse. Suddenly I am shy of telling such a secret as this and wonder darkly if I was only waiting in the wings with these pages in my hands to snatch my uncle's life for my recitative. But some way I feel compelled to tell this tale.

So this is what my uncle told my father and eventually my mother told me: that once during lovemaking, when Henry leaned over to kiss the woman of the night as she lay on the bed, and she rose up to meet him, suddenly it was not her beautiful, perfect face against the pillow but the face of his mother rising up to meet him. Not dead after all, but risen from the grave reproachful as ever, and how it had shocked and staggered him, how he'd paid the woman off and rushed her out of the room, how he had sat in the chair by the bed with his head in his hands, he could not get into that bed again, how he'd had to change hotels. Did you love me, Mother? Did you ever love me? Alfreda's face was as noncommittal as ever. My uncle's loyalty to her was absolute.

And how, ever after, he could only make love to black women.

My uncle had had a black wet nurse, as did my father. He and my father had a mammy. It was just the way of things in the Deep South when they were growing up as Preacher's Kids. And in many essential ways the South had never left him. You could hear it when he spoke, if you listened for it, in the softening at the edges of his words. My uncle—who harbored those deep but subtle racial resentments, a bitter legacy from his Southern past, despite an equally strong sense of social justice—could now only make love to black women. It is a fact so revelatory, so full of human desire and pain, I cannot help but write it down. Maybe original sin is art after all. Once the truth is beheld it ought to be kept secret, yet it must be told. Then again, maybe this is only sophistry after all. What are family stories for but to bear witness to lives that would have otherwise gone silent and unknown? Besides, there was no one on this earth to be shocked by any of it now.

But it's Faulkner all over again. Or Flannery O'Connor. What it says of his misogyny and racism is appalling, I know. But it tells another story to my heart. Something dark, for certain, but also so full of light and insight I can't help but claim it as my own. So it becomes the story of his fragility—the money and the careful use of condoms saving him from his own broken heart. The beautiful black woman in his bed, whom he liked above all others, redeemed him some-how of the mantle of intolerance he now and then so shamelessly wore.

She would be taut, lean, with generous breasts, tawny and smooth, but darkly exotic against the white sheets, his white chest and arms. She would be playful, intelligent, could tell a good joke, laugh in a way that said she really thought he was funny. A quasi relationship. They would have their private name for it. She'd make him feel like he was her favorite, that she couldn't wait for him to come to her again.

Their arms and legs are tangled in a chiaroscuro of black and white. What is this? Sex paid for, yet intimate as the soul's whisper. Flesh of my flesh, my body broken for you. When she moans and shouts *oh God!* for one hundred dollars an hour, he knows she doesn't mean it, but it's all right. It's a fantasy he can hold on to for the appointed hour. When he shouts her name, or *oh god* himself, it's for real, and in that moment, he loses himself in the body of another, in the body of the Other. We are our most vulnerable selves when we are making love. We are opened up to the currents of life. *La petit mort.* The little death. And so he gives himself over, spills himself into the condoms of all false loves, for this one precious hour. *Please don't take your heart from me. Please don't take your heart from me.*

Touch me, touch me please. If I shut my eyes and you touch me like that, just like that, and you pretend you love me it will be enough. Pretend I'm the one you waited for. How splendid this gift from the universe. How bleak and unforgiving to be without it.

He told my father these things, my father who had been faithful to one woman, who pleasured my mother every time. How they loved it, how secret they kept it but for my mother's telling it to me. She was worth a thousand women of the night. To make love to one woman your whole life and never run out of new and wondrous ways to love her, her body familiar and new every time. How my uncle had wanted what my father had always had. Two brothers, twins. A living embodiment of the contradictions in us all. Bright and dark sides of the same thing.

Once in a restaurant some years ago, something happened I hadn't understood until now. We were in Spokane for a visit and out to dinner with the threesome, sometime after my father's stroke. My uncle is busy helping my father with his walker and so he doesn't immediately see the couple sitting in a booth by the window, a white man and a beautiful black woman, something you didn't see every day in conservative Spokane, Washington. I quickly maneuver my uncle into a seat with his back to the couple in the booth behind us and hope for the best. I'm sitting facing them and watch how she touches his wrist, he touches her hand. I do not want any comments or angry stares from my uncle, but he's seen them anyway. He's turned around and looking and we brace ourselves for the biting comment loud enough for anybody to hear. But it never comes. That kind of staring would seem unpardonable, except for the way my uncle's face strangely softened, or so it seems to me now, after what my mother has told me. Then he turns quietly back around and is silent for the rest of the meal.

Now the secrets best left in the dark have been let go. I have yielded to that pull toward story and my desire to see it shape itself into understanding. It's only what I have wondered all along. How human in our frailties we are in the end, so much an alchemy of body and soul.

Three Long Days

The phone rings early one morning. It's the first week of December, 1999. The twins and my mother have been crossed over to safety for two months now, and I have let my guard down. No stairs, no ice or snow, no falling down anymore. It's my mother. "Your father's having a problem," she begins, in her usual, understated way. A problem could be a blood sugar drop, a fall, maybe only a cold. Yet my mind rushes like always straight to death.

"They're taking him to the hospital now. I just wanted you to know." No request for help, although I'm already gathering up my clothes before I hang up the phone. "What happened?" I can barely whisper into the phone.

"He fell in the bathroom."

"But what's wrong?" I am breathless. It feels like my heart has stopped.

"I don't know," she says sharply.

"Are you going with Dad in the ambulance or do you want me to come and get you?" She wishes the latter. She'll postpone the inevitable for as long as possible. I recognize her little dipsy-do. When Grape was dying and they called my mother in the middle of the night to tell her, she said to my father, "I can't go to the hospital now. I have to wash my hair." Pulled out of sleep like that you might say anything. It was that rush back to safety she was after. Then she snapped to. "Is she *in extremis*?" Yes. All right. She would be right down.

By the time I get to my parents' apartment the ambulance has already taken my father away. My uncle is waiting at the door. His voice is hoarse. His eyes are trembling and wide. I help my mother on with her coat. My uncle will wait by the phone. He has come to accept this place by the phone, knowing by then that in a hospital setting he's a terror to himself as well as to others. We all think he's had another stroke but do not say the words. Now it begins.

There are no windows here. Or in any ER room I have ever seen. A window would remind you of the world you've left, the world, by God, you were going to get back to no matter what. A TV bolted to the ceiling in the corner, unspeakable metal things on trays and hanging from the walls, monitors, cuffs, tubes, drawers, cupboards, a metal waste can, all of which in its own time you'd be grateful for if you were thinking straight, instead of hunkered down in some foxhole of your fears. There's a chair for my mother, while I sit on the ledge next to the bed where my father lies pinioned, as we wait for tests to be given, tests to be interpreted, and people in green floating in and out of the room, saying things without comfort and nothing you could hold on to.

Then a terrifying beeping from the heart monitor or maybe the IV drip. If the glucose drip is empty, heart-stopping air must be going into his veins, and no one is rushing in to save him—and even when I learn this is not possible, I cannot stop my rushing heart when that sound splits the air.

I thought everybody was watched over by someone whose only job was to catch these things. But not so. It's a godless universe down here or God gone to sleep at the switch or no God at all. And now the blood pressure readings, too high, too high, 180 over 90 high, spiking whenever he moves or says even a word or two. And a pulse way too slow to keep up with it all. The beeping won't stop. There is no one to stop it. My father keeps looking at the numbers and looking at the door. My mother is only looking at my father. The sound fills the room. I should go out and find someone but I can't move.

"You're tense," my mother says to him with a calm like no other. "That's why your blood pressure is so high." I wonder for a moment what my blood pressure is. And now these funny little hiccoughs in my heart. I can't stand to watch that monitor any longer and I can't look away.

The clack and clamor of metal against metal, bodies floating down the hall on gurneys wheeled perilously around corners, the soft scuttle of shoes against the linoleum, beepings, screeches, moans. I pull up the pale green hospital gown that keeps slipping off my father's shoulders and tuck the thin white blanket under his chin. And then I run away. I do not see all the other broken souls in the other rooms I pass on my way outside. There ought to be windows. There ought to be windows at the very least.

Suddenly I remember how the rain had turned to snow outside the window where I'd waited fifteen years ago in this very same hospital. I'm hunched down into the chair, waiting for my husband to come back from a ghastly surgery I could hardly name. He's gone so far I think he's never coming back. Out the window someone has written *I love you* in the snow on the rooftop below. I sit there for a long time, watching the snow bury the message on the rooftop. You can still see it faintly when they finally wheel him in on a gurney, groggy as hell, but not enough to stop him from kissing me back when I lean over him.

Just two weeks earlier during Christmas at my parents' house in Spokane, we were making love and I reached down to touch him and there it was.

"What's that?" I'd said.

"Oh, that." He turned back over. He knew what I meant.

"I've never felt that before."

"It's always been like that," he said, reaching to take my hand away. He knew all too well where my medical terrors would lead. "You think everything's cancer, and it never is."

Then I turned from him and thought of it as betrayal, not to keep track of such things.

But it was cancer after all, and it had spread. And for a time our lives became thick with a waiting grief—and our lovemaking freighted with death. But that was years ago, and we'd long since crossed over to safety. Except that now, in this very same hospital, here I am again, as frightened as ever.

As frightened as that three-year-old self in an Illinois hospital, with pneumonia in both lungs. My parents can hardly speak of that time, so I know little of the actual sequence of events, except that they were told I might die. What I do remember is screaming as the nuns held me down and gave me shot after bone-aching shot—every three hours night and day for seven days—fifty-eight shots in all, which saved my life, but left me forever terrified in hospitals, or doctors' offices, or near anything metal and sharp and smelling of alcohol.

I'm in the way out here next to the ambulance that has just pulled up and don't want to see the hapless soul rushed through those sliding glass doors. I look up at a faultless sky. Then I go back inside. I'll get a drink, use the bathroom, try my cell phone in the lobby. Then I'll find my way to the cafeteria, get something to eat, bring something for my mother, try to ease my way back in there. But I don't. I rush to my father's room instead. I've been gone too long as it is.

Funny how lately I'd wanted the chance to be alone with my parents without my uncle, funny how this was not what I had in mind. I'd wanted to reminisce, talk about things in earnest. But I sit here unable to speak and so can contribute nothing to the passage of time, and no one's comic relief. Looking at my father stretched out like that so afraid, and my mother stoic and silent too, settling in for the long haul, I just want to cry and cry.

Then the diagnosis at last. Urinary tract infection. Atrial fibrillation. Dehydration. How could he get dehydrated sitting in his easy chair all day? But when you have to take diuretics like he does, dehydration is no trick at all. They will wait to see if the heart rhythm settles down. Otherwise they will shock it back into behaving. That will require sedation, other things.

By the next evening my father is ready to go. He's been rehydrated, his heart-beat is steady, and the antibiotics are starting to kick in. It's dark and rainy and the fog has settled in when Ed and I pick them up at the hospital and bundle my father into the car, my husband and the attendant helping him into his seat, buckling him in tight.

But getting him back out of the car is another matter entirely. He can barely support his weight. And so we grab a wheelchair and roll him up to the apartment. Now he is home. Home from that terrible place.

"Dad, you're home now," I can't help saying out loud.

"Oh," he says, "I never want to go back there again."

Another getaway. Another escape from the treacheries of that place. We ease him into his chair, take off his coat, first the right sleeve, then the left. The right arm always hurts doing this, if you forget to go slow—a side effect of the stroke no one has ever been able to explain.

And then he notices. "Oh my," my father says. Just beyond the cuff of his sweater, there it is: the needle from the IV still tucked neatly into his vein, held down by transparent tape. They'd disconnected the tubing but had forgotten to remove the needle.

The idea of getting him back into the car and driving all the way across town to the hospital is unthinkable. My father puts his head back and shuts his eyes. "I don't want to go back there."

"Well, how hard can this be?" my husband says. I'm thinking of blood spurting all over the front of him, on the walls, the carpet, 911, a tourniquet maybe, the dam unplugged. I can't keep any of this to myself. My husband just looks at me, rolls his eyes. Then he presses down on the vein a couple of inches up from the needle. And slips it out easy as can be, no tugging, no wincing, no trick at all.

"Thank you, Ed," my father says. "I don't ever want to go back there."

The next morning my mother calls again. She's as cool as before. My father has been taken to the hospital again. She gives no details. I rush right over.

"Did your mother tell you about her hand?" my uncle says in a shaky voice, as he opens the door.

"What about her hand?" I say.

A lot has happened already this morning. My uncle has taken over my father's role, stepped into it without missing a beat.

"Mom?" I say. She comes into the living room with a bloody dishtowel around her hand. Her skin is so fragile a whole layer on the top has been peeled away. There is blood everywhere. It's impossible to tell whose blood is whose.

All she can say is, "I might need stitches."

The door to the bloody scene in the bathroom is shut. My father had gone in to use the bathroom, my mother holding on to his belt to steady him, as she had been taught. He was standing there waiting to relieve himself when suddenly he shoots blood all over the bathroom and begins to fall and my mother reaches out to catch him and hits her hand on something and now she's bleeding too, and there is so much blood on everything she doesn't know she's cut herself until they finally take my father away.

So I drive my mother down after the ambulance. She sees a doctor first, before they let her in to see my father. I go in to check on him.

"Hi, Dad," I say.

"I was bleeding everywhere," he says, still astonished that such a thing had happened. "Your mother hurt herself."

"They're fixing her up right now. She's going to be fine." And it turns out they couldn't even give her stitches, the skin on the top of her hand was so thin. They just bandaged it up and said it would heal itself. I think of my mother and her heroic efforts to save my father from falling in all ways, and how fragile she is herself, though she would never admit to it.

"I'm so much trouble," my father says with a sigh. "I didn't want to come back here."

"I know," I say. "But they fixed you up before."

But as it turns out, they'd also damaged him. The nurse, putting in the catheter, had nicked his urethra, and he'd been bleeding ever since.

"She couldn't get it in, and she just kept jabbing me and jabbing me. I told her she was hurting me. But she just kept at it. She said, 'This doesn't really hurt.'"

I had not witnessed this. For such a procedure the daughter was banished to the hall. But oh, the final indignity—if not to the body then to the spirit—was not being believed. And by the time he'd shot blood all over the bathroom, he was already in need of a blood transfusion. And a blood transfusion for my father was by no means a simple thing. Not just a matter of holding your arm still for an hour or so. The increased blood volume spikes the blood pressure, so you take a diuretic, but then run the risk of dehydration again. He's so fragile now, one system so interwoven with the others, he is a lacework of capillaries and veins and pathways in and out.

Finally my father is put into a regular hospital room for the night, and I take my mother home. When we get back to the apartment, she sees that the bathroom is sparkling clean. The blood sprayed all over the toilet and the wall, the bloody, wet towels my mother and uncle had used to try to clean things up, all gone, all gone—and a stack of fresh, clean white towels in their place. Donna, the manager of the dining room and of pretty much everything else at The House, had it all cleaned up, so we wouldn't have to clean it up.

Back at the hospital the next day, some things have been set right. Other things have been discovered: a dangerously low platelet count, a new manifestation of the bone marrow failure discovered several years before the stroke, which explains the profound bleeding. But finally, late the next afternoon, he can finally go home. My parents are going to take a cab. But he will have to go home with the catheter in place, and my mother will have to change the bladder bag. For three days she will have to do this, before they finally send out a visiting nurse to remove it.

But I will not have them going home in some cab. I know what those cab rides can be like. Some of the cab drivers have been in no better shape than my father. The bladder bag, the tubing, and my mother helping to get my father out of the cab all on her own? No. I'll pick them up after work.

I accompany my parents as the nurse wheels my father down to the main floor and into a cold and drafty exit, where, after I get my car, I will park to pick them up. It's after hours and dark and rainy, so when I pull out from the parking lot across from the hospital and into the street I get turned around, and suddenly I am lost. All I can think of is my father huddled against the wind in his thin coat with that bladder bag he's holding in his lap. They're waiting for me at some special night exit, which I have never seen before and now cannot find. I try to retrace my steps but find myself on a street I do not recognize and lose the hospital entirely. By this time I'm beginning to cry and that's not helping me to think, which is what I need to do to find my way back to them.

Eventually I find the hospital again and suddenly recognize the emergency entrance, where I have been twice before, and run in and ask for help. "I can't find my parents," I say in tears. "They're waiting in some kind of special night exit." Oh yes. They know where I need to go. I ask them to repeat the directions because I can't see what they're talking about at all. The words don't even go into my head. All I know is that I have lost them. It was my job to keep them safe and now they are lost. I try frantically to see it all laid out, the right turn, the left turn, but it's a huge medical complex covering several blocks, and street names mean nothing to me, and west and east and north and south mean nothing either.

I get back in my car, say a prayer, which is nothing more than *please*, and then I drive right to them. I'm so glad to see them I burst into tears. I apologize for the delay, and my father says, "That's okay, don't feel bad." My mother is completely silent. She's wondering how she will ever manage all this bladder equipment when they get home, but I don't even think about that right now.

"It's okay," my father says again, "we haven't been waiting long." The nurse, who's been waiting with them, just looks at me. We get my father out of the wheelchair and edge him over to the passenger seat of the van and untangle the tubing that runs out of him into the bladder bag, which we put safely by his feet in the well of the car, then we're on our way. It does not occur to me that I will eventually have to get him out of the car. My only thought is finding my way home in the dark.

How I manage to get us home in that sleety rain I do not know. But somehow I intuit my way down the hill, to a freeway entrance going north. The rest of the way I know by heart. Then there it is at last, the high, white building rising up out of the night. University House. The purple awning, the lighted doors that will glide open to greet us, the lobby with the Chihuly glass. I rush inside and get the wheelchair loaner from the storeroom. I position the wheelchair as close to the car as I can and reach in to help him out of the seat. But he's almost dead weight by now. His foot gets all tangled up in the catheter tubing. He leans back against the seat as I untangle it. Then I hand the catheter bag to my mother, who's having a hard time herself, keeping the bag close to him, because there isn't enough tubing for a long extension. I'm afraid he'll slip from my arms and fall to the pavement, or miss the wheelchair altogether, or hit it halfway and flip it over. If I can just get my arms under him and hold him up while he takes a step and swivels from the seat of the van down to the seat of the waiting wheelchair.

"Dad, can you help me a little?"

"I'll try. I'm just so weak."

It takes every bit of strength and balance I've got and some I haven't to get him the single step from the car into the wheelchair. But I do it. I am trembling from the effort. I do not think of calling for help. It doesn't occur to me that there is any help for us in the universe. In that moment it's just my father and me and my mother holding the bladder bag in the slanting rain.

The next day when I stop by just to see how the night went, I pull up to the front of the building and shudder at the scene with the wheelchair the night before. I haven't even turned off the engine when an aid car rushes around the corner and pulls in right in front of me. I could sit in my car and count to twenty and tell myself that this frantic aid car could be for anybody. Over three hundred people live here and it could be for any one of them. Or I could rush after the two guys dashing inside now with their bags and defibrillators. And I do. But they turn the corner and disappear into the elevator before I can catch up.

The woman at the desk stops me. Of course I know what she wants. She wants to say don't go up there! You don't want to see it. I can't breathe. I stand at the desk and see spots before my eyes. My vision is closing in. I turn around and look at the sun shining through the windows, on the big pots of yellow and blue flowers rippling in the breeze, the dark purple awning. I want to run out of here and into the sun. I wouldn't even have to get in my car and drive away. I could just stand there with the sun on my shoulders, my face, and close my eyes.

"Here. You forgot to sign in," the woman at the desk says petulantly. "You need to sign in when you come here."

You bitch, I say to myself. *You goddamned bitch.*

But I understand. My parents are relatively new here, and apparently so am I. I pick up the pen and write my name. But when I look I see I've written my maiden name. I've written *Ann Cunningham*. Right then I am my father's daughter and no one else. Everything slows down, except my heart.

Then I'm standing in front of the elevators unable to push the button. Suddenly the doors snap open and a woman walks out. No disasters are written on her face. She's wearing a red coat and stylish black hat, black gloves, ready for an outing to the ballet or symphony. I remember her rouged cheeks and bright lips. I envy her freedom, her sense of herself. I think of my mother's face beautiful without makeup, think of her bandaged right hand, her skin too fragile even for stitches, and wish for her a better life. I can't imagine what all this would have been like if it had happened to her three hundred miles away from me—and I step into the elevator at last.

But it's all right. The ambulance wasn't for him, at least not this time.

And the phone. Everything about it changed after those three days. To see my parents' name on the caller ID was terrifying to me. "Your father is having a problem." Yes, as it turned out, he was having problems of one kind or another all the time now. So many things were going wrong. Yet my parents, or rather my mother, tried very hard not to call for just anything, but to wait for the check-in call I made every night. So whenever I saw that they had called, or saw who it was as the phone was ringing, my hands grew cold before I even picked up the phone.

"Hi, Mom. I saw that you called. What's up?"

"We've just called 911. They're on their way." Or the truly terrifying, the call from my uncle. "They've just taken your father to the hospital. Your mother went with him in the ambulance."

But once in a while, once every blessed while, I forced myself to listen to the message before my frantic fingers dialed the phone. And there it was. My mother's stilted voice on the answering machine:

"Hello. This is your mother. Please add two four-packs of toilet paper to the grocery list. Thank you."

Yes, thank you thank you thank you. It was only toilet paper after all. But when the phone rang it was death every time and never toilet paper at all. I came to hate the phone. Hated talking on the phone, hated the ringing of the phone. At my desk or with students, it would ring behind my back, startling me into a heart-pounding, breathless moment it was taking me increasingly longer to ease out of. And later his collapse while Ed and I were at our little mountain cabin by the Naches River and completely out of phone range, just to remind us not to go too far. I was tethered to them now, bound by invisible wires across the miles.

Or his collapse the night before I was to leave for a stay at a writer's colony. I'd been chosen out of hundreds of applicants for a three-week stay in one of six cottages at Hedgebrook Writers Colony on Whidbey Island, west of Seattle. I would go there where nothing was asked of me but to write. A writer can only go there once, and this was my chance. I didn't know if my heart was ready or if I had my fair share of courage. So I'd wanted to get ready meditatively, deliberately, gather my strength for the writing journey that lay ahead.

Now it was one in the morning and I'd been at the hospital all evening, though finally they were moving my father out of the ER up to a bed on the sixth floor. I was sitting in a little side room filling out a form about my father's bowel habits for the charge nurse. My mother was exhausted. "You do it," she said. "Just make it up." After all, I was a fiction writer. They'd find out soon enough what was what. That splendid cottage in the woods, the stained glass windows, the hardwood floors, the window seat for reading, the bedroom loft, gourmet meals brought to my doorstep, the forest all around. And the hours lined up one after the other for uninterrupted writing. I would be like Thoreau. I could go to the woods. Or I could stay with my father in this hospital.

But my mother said, "You have to go. We'll be all right." And so I left my father and went to the woods. I spent three weeks writing in that cottage with stained glass windows and hardwood floors, expecting any day another phone call to draw me back into that other life I had left behind.

Heart irregularity, urinary tract infection (again), foot infection (they might have to amputate), bronchitis (again), side effects from the previous ER visit, bone marrow failure, platelet drop, prostate cancer (treatable with Luprin shots), diabetes, strange things that could not be named. So many reasons to call.

Appointment with the Dark

And now so many doctors, so many appointments, so many cab rides to the cardiologist, urologist, dermatologist, gerontologist, oncologist, hematologist, endocrinologist. My mother and I used to laugh and say the only one my father hadn't seen yet was the gynecologist. Then we'd joke about my father after his appendectomy years ago.

"Grace," he'd said more times than she could count. "They *had* to have taken out more than my appendix. It hurts too much."

"Yes, Homer," she says, "you're right. They also took out your uterus."

But with each new complication, a new specialist and the question: Will you be the last one? Will you be the doctor who helps see him out? All were part of the Virginia Mason Medical Center in downtown Seattle, connected by breezeways to Virginia Mason Hospital. Dr. Johnston, the cardiologist, whose photography on the walls my father admired, was a lovely, white-haired man who called my father *Dr.* Cunningham. They discussed favorite kinds of cameras, since my father had been a photographer too. He made my father feel like a person. "Heart failure," he said as gently as he could. We were stunned. But his heart was always the strongest part of him. Dr. Johnston prescribed a new combination of pills that fixed it, more or less, for the moment. And then he retired. So he wouldn't be the last doctor after all. The urologist, whose name I never knew, whom I had never met, as I waited decorously in the waiting room, as any good daughter would do, wouldn't be the one either. Dr. Gross, the endocrinologist, must have been teased as a child with a name like that, but he was a large man who'd probably been able to fend for himself, or so I hoped, because he was so kind to my father and so thorough. He was new to the clinic and far from any thought of retirement. He kept track of my father's blood sugars and insulin dosages, and I hoped he would be the last one.

Dr. Featherston was my father's gerontologist and primary care physician. She was a large woman with long dark hair streaked with gray, who'd taken some kind of leave herself, who told my mother, when my father had slept through his exam, "He really belongs in a nursing home now." And my mother reported this to me with such heartbreak and anguish I knew it was true. We did everything we could not to believe in this. But we knew my father was in a new place now, somewhere between one thing and another. We could go on like this forever, I thought. It's not so bad. But as it turned out, it was my mother who could not.

Soon I would be leaving for Cuba again, to give a paper at a Hemingway conference. It felt farther away than ever. No phone calls to Cuba now, no emergency flights home, for Cuba was as forbidden to Americans then as it is today. No phone wires could connect us now. I asked Dr. Featherston if she thought my father would be all right while I was gone. I would only be gone ten days. I wanted her to say, "Sure, go ahead, you can't put your life on hold for what might happen. He'll be all right." But she didn't.

"You must know he's on a slippery slope," she said, a little impatiently. I had followed her into her office without invitation. That slippery slope talk would not be enough for me. "What do you mean, exactly?" I said, standing my ground.

"He's *old!* He's eighty-six years old. Everything's wearing out."

"I know," I said. "But I wouldn't leave if . . ." I couldn't finish my thought. She just looked at me.

He'd been on a slippery slope since that Friday morning three years ago when he'd slipped off the chair onto the floor.

But my mother said "Go," and so I did.

My father had been diagnosed with a disorder of the bone marrow a few years before his stroke, which went without a precise name for a long time. It was not cancer, but cancerlike. At first it affected his production of red blood cells, and so he carried the weight of a great fatigue for a long time. He slept a lot in his chair, and looked pale most of the time. Then with the profound bleeding in December, two months after they had moved to Seattle, my father was referred to a hematologist for further workup. He ordered a bone marrow test, which was never an easy procedure, and whose results we were to receive on this, our first visit. His name was Vincent Picozzi, and he was the doctor we came to know the best. With all of my father's problems, the most profound was this one of the bone marrow.

The waiting room of a hematology/oncology office is designed for a long, anxious wait. I remember the coffee urn and the water cooler, for those waiting their turn alone, or with some devoted family member. The fish tank for the bald children and their astonished mothers, where fish floated in a cool blue sea, divided one side of the room from the other. Though there was no official designation, one side of the fish tank seemed to be for *the sick* and the other, the left side, for *the very sick*—that is, those with no hair, who wore white face masks to screen out any germs carried in by people who'd missed the sign on the front wall: NO GERMS ALLOWED. ALL THOSE WITH COUGH OR FLU KEEP OUT! More or less. A wall of windows on the side of *the very sick* looked out over the city, and on lucky days, you could see the sun shimmering on Lake Union in the distance. I stood there often, looking out at the sun on the water and imagined myself anyplace but here.

The handicapped bathroom was on the right side of the fish tank, and we always sat conveniently close to it because the wait was always so long, and my father invariably had to use it, which was another ordeal my mother excused me from. She would wheel him in and shut the door behind her. My job was to guard the door, to stand just outside and listen for any calls for help from within. How she did all this on her own, before she assented to my offers of help, I do not know. Though this was one of the ways they were intimate now, these bathroom trips that excluded everyone else. That there might have also been tenderness in those times and not just trouble, I can only hope.

But eventually our name would be called—that is, *Homer Cunningham's* name would be called—and I would push the wheelchair through the double doors into the inner sanctum while my mother followed close behind and down the busy hall into the examining room, where we would wait for another long stretch of time.

Dr. Picozzi himself was not an attractive man. You not only excused this but it comforted you somehow. He was so earnest and so busy in the lab with all his patients' protocols he never had time to get to the mall, probably wasn't married and so had no wife to keep him in shape, or get him to a decent barber. Or perhaps it was the arduous nature of his job—where many of his patients did not get better—that took its toll on whatever good looks he might have originally had. It was surely a face best suited for the lab.

On this day, our first, Dr. Picozzi introduces himself and sits down on the doctor's stool and begins to look over the papers in the manila folder with my father's name on it, and since they had forwarded all my father's records, it was a long read, which included the blood taken just an hour ago. So we've nothing to do but watch him scan my father's reports. He's sitting there in his white lab coat, his thin, striped cotton shirt gaping at the buttonholes across his middle, his tight polyester pants rising above his socks, and today, partially unzipped from the strain. I study his dark-haired comb-over and wonder at this sad concession to vanity, while my father keeps his precarious balance on the end of the examining table.

Dr. Picozzi looks up and, having read that my father had been a history professor, begins quizzing him about the Civil War, while we wait anxiously for the results of my father's bone marrow test he's holding in the manila folder in his hands, which strikes my mother and me as somewhat bizarre. I look at my father, hunched over now from the strain of keeping his balance. He's always all dressed up for these appointments; my mother makes sure of that—his camel blazer with the suede elbows, his blue shirt to add some color to his pale complexion, his brown oxfords. Anything to convince the doctor that this man is worth saving. Please don't throw him away.

Dr. Picozzi asks my father questions about the Battle of Antietam, which of course my father knows. I think it's more the doctor showing off than making the patient feel at home, although it might not seem that way if you didn't go into every doctor's appointment with suspicion and automatic mistrust. Then a darker thought occurs to me. This isn't doctor-patient bonding. This is a mental test. And a way to see if my father's life is worth his time and this new and staggeringly expensive treatment he's about to propose. Is there still quality of life here? Is this man still worth saving? This is grossly unfair I am sure, but I felt it nevertheless.

I tried very hard to feel warm toward Dr. Picozzi, my father's last doctor, or so I thought, to echo my father when he said what a good doctor he was, something he practically always said now about his doctors, to feel he was being kept safe and not in harm's way in this place that had so surely traumatized him in that first visit to the ER.

So finally, after Picozzi delivers the verdict—a failure of the bone marrow to produce red blood cells, and now a failure to produce enough platelets, and thus the profound bleeding from the nick in the ER weeks ago—my father asks, "Am I ready to kick the bucket?"

"Well," Picozzi says. He's clearly startled that this question had come so abruptly and in such a fashion.

"How long have I got?" my father repeats.

"How long do any of us have? How long do I have?" Picozzi says, looking everywhere but at my father. "If you mean, does this diagnosis," what it was could not be named exactly, "will it shorten your life? I don't know. Maybe. We don't really know." A studied, practiced answer, and very useful over the years, I imagine, given the harrowing field he was in, where many did not survive.

Then Dr. Picozzi gives us just what we have come all this way for. Dr. Picozzi gives us the possibility of a miracle. A seven-thousand-dollar-a-month miracle called the EPO shot. It was such a new therapy it was just this side of experimental. The EPO did not work on everyone, of course, but it was worth a good solid try.

That day of bad news and good news was all too much—the forty-minute drive to their apartment, the cab ride downtown with them, the wheelchair, the handicapped bathroom, the ghastly wait, the Civil War questions, the verdict, the bald children. I thought of their tenuous, otherworldly lives. My father was eighty-six, and as precious to me as he had ever been. Still, if one had to choose between my father and one of those children, of course, life owed *them* the miracles. I didn't know what it still owed my father.

After our appointments at the medical center, my parents would then "take me out to lunch," in the hospital cafeteria, a place that never failed to fill me with dread. If you were in hospital greens, you were just on your lunch break. But street clothes meant something else altogether. I wondered how much sorrow and fear that busy cafeteria held at lunchtime. Eventually you would have to eat, no matter how long you'd been keeping watch in a hospital room.

Soon we're all situated at a table that can accommodate my father's wheelchair, though it's a tight fit between the wheelchair and the table across the aisle.

We've skipped the hot food service entirely—unidentifiable things floating in grease—macaroni and cheese, lasagna, meatballs mired in a slick, gray gravy. I never have understood it—such unhealthy food in a hospital. No wonder so many folks in hospital greens have brought their own lunch in Tupperware containers or brown sandwich bags. I didn't learn until several years later, when my mother was hospitalized, what this was all about. "We want people to eat, above all," a nurse told me. "Fat and salt stimulate their appetites." And I suppose eating this stuff is better than not eating at all.

Then I've got everybody's tray of food and my father is working on a ham sandwich and a bowl of clam chowder. My mother's nibbling at half a turkey sandwich and that's all. I'm tackling a salad and a Diet Pepsi.

Then in a voice loud enough to be heard across the aisle, my father says: "That man over there," he says, pointing to an older man with a graying crew cut. "He's a GI and that's his Korean war bride." And I look at them, the man with a patient ID bracelet on his wrist, navy windbreaker, the wife across the table, diminutive and quiet, her dark shiny hair, and I think he's probably right. But of course right now I'm not generous enough to say anything like that.

So I tell him: "Don't *say* things like that. They'll hear you."

"But I like to watch people. I like to imagine their lives."

I'm ashamed I spoke so sharply. It pains me now to remember how sharply it had come out. What do writers do anyway, but imagine other people's lives? To my great discredit, I had only chided an old man who'd lost his sense of context and propriety. I was worn out by this doctor's visit. I was angry that my father had grown so old, that he would die and probably soon now, and that I couldn't do anything to stop it. Yet if I was exhausted, what about him? The visit had not been wonderful. He had been given the results of a painful bone marrow test and learned grave and despairing news, and then the wrenching possibility of hope.

"I'm just impedimenta," he says, as I'm wheeling him out of the hospital and down to the lobby to wait for the cab.

"Don't *say* that," I repeat. "And don't say you're a *cripple* either." He looks like I've slapped him.

"Okay," he says softly. "But that's the way I feel."

He was only saying what he felt, and we could not abide it. We could not admit it by day, and only whispered it in the night, in the secret self that mourned the loss of him and the losses to come. But he was all these things. No. His body was all these things. I don't think he ever understood the tenderness we felt in caring for him. How we felt his spirit by touching his body.

Poor Dr. Picozzi.

"So how do you feel, Mr. Cunningham?" he asked after this therapy had begun. It's *Dr.* Cunningham, I wanted to add, but of course I didn't want to piss him off.

"About the same," my father said, usually so weary by then of the wait for the blood work that always preceded these visits, the transport up two floors to Hematology and then the inevitable waiting in that office—that he could not put on a good face for it, though for so long he tried to kid his doctors, show he had some spunk left, that he himself was still there.

And later still, Dr. Picozzi would sit holding my father's lab results in the file he held before him so thrilled with the numbers on the page. The expensive, experimental shot was working, theoretically anyway, though my father reported no increase in energy, and still had that devastating fatigue. And then came the platelet crisis for which there was no treatment, no monthly seven-thousand-dollar shot—only periodic blood transfusions, which carried their own particular risk of blood pressure spikes and diuretic-induced dehydration.

Still, I hoped Dr. Picozzi would not be my father's last doctor. Dr. Picozzi was not the one you'd want sitting by the bed holding your hand, though you would surely want him in the lab finding a cure. But he'd been able to pull the proverbial rabbit out of the hat, for which I excused him all his awkwardness, the dismissive way he treated my father, the way he ignored my mother and me, how he talked to the air and not to us. What did he know about people anyway, growing up in a petri dish?

Later there were other doctors, but none we would remember. And his last doctor was someone we never met, who in all probability had never met my father, who collected the Medicare checks and signed off on the prescriptions. There was no doctor in the end, no doctor to see him out.

And so we all went on with our lives as best we could, and with each complication a little less of him returned. Then came the strange aches and pains, the mysterious nausea, the pain in his right shoulder and arm I'd hoped was a sign of a resurrection of the nerves that had died. But no, it was just ordinary pain and no miracle at all.

And the sudden, garbled speech. He'd wake in the morning to find another part of him had flown off in the night. Then by evening the sentences would start out just fine but fall apart after a few seconds. And then his astonishment more than panic that the sounds did not quite match up with his thoughts, like a film with the sprockets out of sync. All evidence of little, undetectable strokes he'd been having all along, that mostly resolved themselves outwardly but took their toll on inner things.

Or the mornings when my mother could not wake him because he had gone someplace far in his sleep and would not be called back until he finally heard her say, "Homer, if you don't wake up, I'm going to have to call 911." So he would eventually rouse himself and assent to being called back to life from wherever he had gone, and the day would begin.

I would visit as often as I could, and we kept our Sunday dinner ritual without fail. Stepping into the lobby of University House cheered me. In the lobby, with the sculptures and the paintings on the walls, you could pretend your parents were on some fabulous holiday, and this was their hotel, or that they lived in some elegant penthouse or condominium. I could keep this feeling going in the elevator with the clean promise of no smell at all, and even down the hallways, but I had to work hard to keep it going as I approached Apartment 320.

Inside my parents' apartment now were most of the accoutrements of the handicapped—the "scooter," the wheelchair, the walker, the cane, the guard rail on my father's bed, the booster seat for the toilet. And now this new smell. So I took a deep breath and paused to gather myself before I knocked on the door. Then I made my entrance with my usual flair, *It's me!* I sang it out with all the enthusiasm I could muster. They so looked forward to my visits and said I always gave them such a "lift," which was gratifying of course, but also struck me with guilt for all the days I had not managed to visit, for all the times I did not stay long enough. A *lift* was something that kept you off the bottom, raised you up. The lift was me. And some days I could not be funny enough or cheerful enough to banish the sadness in that room or keep it from gathering in the corners of my eyes. And worse, that feeling of claustrophobia, that unspeakable feeling that I couldn't wait to leave. That's how those visits were, the last months they were all together, I am ashamed to admit, because I would give anything now to have them back.

My beautiful uncle, my elegant bachelor uncle, wore diapers now. The diapers were the ignominious side effect of the prostate surgery he'd had ten years ago, and the moment that marked the beginning of his giving up on life. It pained me to see the bulk in the rear of his brown pants, shiny from wear, as he walked across the room. He didn't notice the odor when he neglected to change them often enough or the way they smelled, stored in the waste can too long. It was the smell of neglect, despair, and coming death. It was the smell of the nursing home, only I didn't know it then. My mother was now putting Floral Glade on her shopping list every week. It embarrassed her and pained her particularly because she knew she must have grown accustomed to it and worried that others would notice that telltale odor before she did.

Sometimes when I visited I would imagine that my father had died, sleeping in that chair slumped to the side, slack-jawed and pale. He'd struggle to open his eyes, just to see that I was still there, smile at me, and then settle back down into a dark and irresistible sleep. My mother called it the Cunningham Curse. "He sleeps all day. No wonder he can't sleep at night." And my father, finally jolted awake by my mother's voice, would say, "I'm not sleeping. I was just resting. I heard everything you said."

Henry had been sleeping all day for years. But his sleeping sickness was of a different order. His was an undiagnosed, untreated, and profound depression. But with my father it was easier to talk of this sleeping as the Cunningham Curse than to reference bone marrow tests, red blood cell counts, a slowing-down heart. But if my father was asleep, my uncle would become suddenly animated, full of jokes, wisecracks. On the rare occasion when my father held forth, my uncle would slip down into sleep in his chair while the conversation went on around him. Then he would wake up as I was putting on my coat to go. "You're leaving? You just got here!" And then my inevitable guilt for not having come sooner or stayed longer or visited more often, the sigh and the deep breath at the door before I came in. The children felt it too, though my husband was exempt from such things.

Yet looking back on it now, there are certain things that gather up my guilt in strange, inexplicable ways. In themselves they are illogical, but they call forth great meaning as metaphor, and in dreams.

The story of the trip to the zoo, which never happened, is one of those things. The zoo was the one place where I most wanted to take my father but never did. I wanted to take him by myself, so it would be just the two of us. My mother and uncle could never have walked it, so I wanted to take my father in his wheelchair some lovely, warm summer day. All our trips now were to the medical center or to and from the hospital, and of course our Sunday dinners out.

My father loved the idea of wild animals and safari hunting. He was a histo-

rian and a scholar and knew mostly inside things. And though he was no fisherman or hunter, he subscribed to *Outdoor Life* and *Field and Stream*. My father
was in love with the adventurous male life he only wished he had. His own father,
J.B. the minister, an inside person too, did no safari hunting either.

To say I spent my early childhood living in attics and college dorms would
take some explaining, but it tells why pets were always problematic for my family.
There were just the three of us, my academic parents and me, living in Greenville,
Illinois, where I was born, first in the boys' dorm when my father was dean of
men until I was three; in a duplex down the street when I was four; then when I
was five, tucked away in a little attic apartment outside New York City while my
father went to NYU; the Greenville College girls' dorm when my mother was
dean of women until I was nine; then a rented house where no pets were allowed
until we moved to Spokane when I was ten. We had few things to carry with us
as we moved from place to place over those years of my childhood. Everything
we needed we already had.

I desperately wanted a dog, though our living circumstances would only
allow small pets you could keep in cages. When I was seven, my father bought me
a chameleon at a little circus that set up tent just outside of our small Illinois college town. I remember the trapeze artist and the lone elephant who went round
and round that sawdust floor. I loved the glamour of the circus, the costumes, the
sequins, the tights, the glittery makeup. Of course, I wanted to join the circus,
which inspired me to organize a neighborhood "circus" that summer, for which
I perfected my most dazzling trick—a no-handed backbend, where I grabbed a
paper cup between my teeth filled with water off the ground, and drank it as I
came back up. I fell in love with show business then, and though my father was
leery of this world, he was responsible for my introduction to it.

My chameleon's gender was never determined, but I named her Maggie
anyway. She did not change color when I placed her on various colors of construction paper. She just skittered off under the couch to my screaming when I

grabbed her by the tail, and it came off in my hand. "That's all right," my father said, "they just grow new ones."

Maggie would not eat chameleon food. She would only eat live flies. So my father went hunting for flies by the garbage cans in the alley out behind the Greenville College dining hall, and collected them in a mayonnaise jar, then shook them into the cage he'd built out of balsa wood and screening for Maggie, who immediately began the pursuit of dinner. My father was so proud of that cage, so perfect and snug, given his limited experience and abilities with tools. And the next year he built me a pair of stilts that had me towering over my friends as I clomped my way around campus.

When it turned fall, my father sat me down on a bench under a blazing elm tree next to the college library, and explained that there would be no flies in winter, and the chameleon needed to be let go into the woods by the lake, where it could make its winter home. My father took the chameleon away and put it somewhere safe in the woods by the lake. I could not bear to go along, and truly, my father seemed relieved. We never talked about where he took it exactly, or its probable fate, or how it could even make a winter home.

When I was eight, I got a baby chick. Instead of bringing cupcakes for the class to celebrate his son's birthday, Freddy Macon's father brought a baby chick for each member of the class. He went around the room and set a little cardboard box on each desk. I stared at it for a minute, listening to the little scratching sound inside, before I opened the top, and there it was. My very own Easter chick. I carried it home in that little cardboard box, walking as slowly as I could manage, though I was so excited I wanted to run all the way home. My parents would be so excited too. Freddy's father owned the only feed store in Greenville, so there was a logic to this gift, because now there were thirty families who had to go to the feed store to buy chicken food.

But the baby chick had to be given away too, when it grew out of its Easter baby chick stage and began to become an actual chicken. My parents and I were living in the Greenville College girls' dorm at the time, so I can only imagine the accommodations my mother and father made to keep a live chicken in my father's study just off my mother's dean of women's office.

When I was nine, Marsha Sanderson, an elderly friend of my parents, gave me a parakeet. When I was ten, I gave it back to her. I'd named him Binky and set his cage by the dining room window next to the piano. He'd chirp and grab the side of the cage with his claws and flap his wings whenever my mother played the piano. I taught him to say *pretty bird* and *pretty Binky* and *howdydoo*. The day before we set off on our trek across the country to our new home in Spokane, I gave him back to Marsha. This time I knew my pet really would have a winter home. This time my parents promised that once we moved to Spokane and had a house of our own, I could finally have a dog, and I would never have to give her away.

Though our family never went camping or even hiking, my childhood was filled with jungle adventures anyway. My father's closest encounter with wild nature was on the seventeenth hole of an Illinois golf course, when he went to reach down to retrieve his ball from the cup. But some preternatural sense stopped him, and he poked his golf club down the hole first. A cottonmouth came boiling out of the hole, as he jumped back and swung his club and killed it. To my father it was divine intervention. The staying of the hand, that split second when you turned left not right, or stepped back just at the moment of impact. Any life has such near misses. But to my father it meant that he was watched over. And that I was too. I'd heard the story enough times to believe it: There was another snake in our family mythology, this one in Pennsylvania when I was three, and playing on Grandpa and Grandma Piper's front porch. I was called back from death moments before a copperhead slithered up onto the porch right where I had been playing a minute before.

My father was a worrier and saw dangers everywhere. Maybe that's why he so loved the idea of danger encountered vicariously, heroically. He would explain which snakes were the most poisonous and where they could be found. He often told me the story of growing up in Florida, where there were plenty of snakes, and of the day in grade school when a kid carried a coral snake to school in his pocket, for show and tell. A coral snake, my father explained, is the most poisonous snake in North America, because it's related to the cobra, which, he assured me, is found only in India. He taught me all about the poisonous snakes of the world, which should have frightened me, but like him, I was fascinated and truly not afraid. I knew that the most poisonous snake in the world was the green mamba, but it was far away in Africa and that was all right. The green mamba, he said, was more poisonous than the coral snake and more poisonous even than the black mamba, which always sounded like the most poisonous snake to me, though he was always quick to point out that none of these snakes lived in New York or Illinois. I knew about cottonmouths though, or the water moccasins, as they were often called, that were supposed to live in the rushes near the shore of the far side of Greenville Lake where we swam each Illinois summer. But these stories didn't frighten me. They thrilled me. They were proof of my providential life, of my uniqueness on this earth.

I loved the snake house at the St. Louis Zoo. I loved watching the snakes all curled up inside their cages, loved standing a Plexiglas inch away from that sleepy danger ready to unwind and strike out in a flash. DON'T TAP ON THE GLASS, the signs read. But of course that's what everybody wanted to do. To see the snake rise up and open its mouth, and lunge at you while you stayed safely in the dark.

My father and I used to watch a TV program together on Sunday afternoons called *Ramar of the Jungle*. It was obvious, even to me, that it was a Hollywood set they were tromping through in their safari jackets and helmets, juxtaposed with what was clearly spliced footage of roaring lions and marauding elephants.

During my kindergarten year when we lived in New York, in that safe, cozy attic, with the sloping ceiling, and the little secret window that looked out over town, I remember waiting Friday nights for my father to come home for the weekend from the his little student apartment on the campus of NYU, and tuck me in and tell me the new *John Stories* he'd made up on the subway coming back from the city. The *John Stories* were always set in Africa, which is an especially dangerous place to be if you are the kind of klutz John was, always falling down or doing goofy, awkward things that set him in the path of danger, but so comically that I was never afraid for him or for me. I was always tripping and dropping things myself, and so I had a special affection for John, who went on safaris and encountered lions and rhinos and elephants and snakes of all kinds. John discovered diamonds and rubies and emeralds, and seemed to be watched over too.

It was no wonder, then, that I would want to take my father to the zoo, since University House, where he lived now, was just ten minutes away. At the zoo we could travel back through time, when we were both whole and there was no sadness or loss in sight, and days upon days of sunlight stretched out before us. If the day were warm and sunlit and not too crowded and he didn't have to use the bathroom suddenly, or get too tired, and his back didn't hurt, we could go for an hour or so before one of these ended our trip.

As it turned out, the only excursions he and I took alone together were in his last days, the ones he spent at the Ida Culver Nursing Home, where he went a year later. The nursing home was attached to the Ida Culver Retirement Home, two worlds joined by a couple of elevator rides and a long, Byzantine hallway. But by then we were in another country, and already as far away as we had ever been. Since I had come to think of the nursing home as a zoo anyway, the jungle metaphor worked in reverse. All the dangerous beasts of the jungle were behind us now, in that other place, as we crossed over to the other side where people lived in relative safety and health.

We'd take the elevator from floor 2, where he lived now, the floor for people like him, who would never be going home, to floor 3, then across the hall to a different elevator, then back down to floor 2 that opened up onto the other side. It was the way you got from one world to another. The elevator on my father's floor carried the earthly smells of death, the other elevator the glorious smell of nothing at all.

"Let's go try to find a soda machine," I say one night, trying to make this as much of an adventure as I can.

"Okay," my father says, flashing me that worried look, "but don't get lost."

Dad, we are already lost, I thought. We are as lost as we can be.

Actually, at that moment, we *are* lost. I'd taken a wrong turn and would not be able to simply reverse our direction to find our way back. "We can't really get lost here," I say, with a laugh that hides the catch in my throat. I want to lean over and put my face against his head. I want to put my arms around him but am afraid I will cry. I want to find the main lobby and just roll him out the front door and keep on going and never come back. But he has no hat or coat and it's a cold, rainy night in early March, and gusts of wind would blow slanting rain in our faces and down our necks.

We pass a man getting into his apartment with a load of groceries.

"Excuse me," I say, "is there a soda machine around here somewhere?"

"Oh," he says, putting down his groceries. "There used to be a soda machine, but they took it out. I don't know why they did that. I always have to buy it at the store." He looks at us again and smiles. You can tell he's sizing us up. But it's clear to anybody that we do not live here.

"Do you know the way back to the nursing home?" my father asks.

The man blinks but continues to smile. This is knowledge he does not want to have.

"Wait right here," he says, and disappears through the door only to return a few moments later with a Coke for each of us. He's so kind, and elderly himself, he must be counting his good fortune to be here and not where we have obviously come from.

"Oh thank you," my father says, recovering a bit of his social grace. He just looks at the man, astonished at this gesture, at his wholeness.

"Yes, thanks so much."

"We can't drink these," my father says, as we roll down the hall.

"I know, but wasn't that nice?"

"We should have said Diet Coke," he says. "We can't have sugar."

"But it was nice anyway."

My father has lost something in the translation. He's forgotten that this kind man was not taking our order. But soon enough my father can have all the regular Coke or anything else he wants. We're only a few weeks away from it, our new gig, the hospice gig, where the only rule is: there aren't any rules anymore.

Was his former life unremembered now? Or remembered beyond bearing, as he rode past door after door with gold-framed nameplates, which said here I am, here I will stay, and little ledges where folks put out flowers or pictures or mementos that said to anyone passing by who they were. My father's door in the nursing home was never closed, though he himself was hidden behind a curtain that often separated his side from his roommate's. The only sense that he was there at all is his name written on a piece of tagboard in black marker, as such things are subject to change.

But soon he'd had enough. "Can we go back now?" my father asks. Of course there's no going back, and on some level he knows it too.

"Sure," I say. "We're not really lost."

He turns and smiles at me and sheds that worried look. "Okay. You're the driver."

Like animals, we could have found our way home with our sense of smell. That sweet, thick, earthy smell of life at its end. But eventually we found the hallways and elevators that led us back to his room and his bed and his TV and his chair. He was worn out and so was I. It would have been better if we'd sat and talked, drinking Diet Cokes I had brought in, remembering John and the lions and elephants and snakes and diamonds.

Lyric from a Thin Place

And so the last year with the threesome passed, with the inevitable falterings of people growing old, pulled both forward and back, yet moving inexorably toward death. The end of my uncle's story began in October 2001, a month after the world as we all knew it changed forever. Death had moved in, but did not announce itself in any way we recognized at the time. It did not ruffle the air or cast shadows across the sunlight that came as unabashed as ever through the windows. Even its whisperings went unheard.

My father had held all the family medical drama for so long that my uncle's travails were eclipsed even now. Uncle Henry had strange and mysterious symptoms, but he'd had a lifetime of these—mysterious aches and pains that came and went, strange feelings of fatigue, dizziness, a malaise outside of words.

But in the two years my uncle lived at University House he had made no trips to the ER, was never hospitalized, could get to his doctor downtown by himself in a cab. Of course the letter he received telling him his pacemaker might be defective hung over him like a "Damocles sword," as he liked to call it. And he was now having weekly blood tests to regulate his Coumadin levels, which he was taking for his syncopating heart. Still, it seemed as though he would easily outlive my father, if you saw the two of them side by side.

Looking back on them now, the last days of my uncle's life were strange and revelatory, if only we had known what was before us. Yet all three had been in that other country for years now. They all seemed on the precipice of near and ever present danger you could only see in between eyeblinks or heartbeats. In recent weeks my uncle had complained about a mysterious pain in his groin that no test could identify. It made it hard for him to walk. Now and then he had taken to using my father's walker. When he pushed my father's wheelchair to dinner those days, something he insisted on regularly now, he was using it as much for himself as for my father. He had taken to using his cane without being reminded. He tripped and fell more frequently and sometimes could not get himself back up, even with the chair my mother scooted over to him and kept steady while he tried to raise himself from the floor.

Sometimes he did not go down to dinner, but had it sent up. Those were the nights my parents were a couple again, and would be seated with other couples, which in the old days would have resulted in new friendships and a fine time. But that could never happen now, as relationships at The House were fragile at best, and the opportunities for such acquaintances so rare. And now and then my uncle would not feel up to our Sunday dinner out, and so it would be the four of us, two couples out on the town.

It was the third week in October, and the light had held a thin, attenuated feel for weeks now. The blue of that October sky felt extravagant and pure for only an hour or two at best, before an uncertainty settled over us, and then faded into dark completely. Soon the time would change and we'd lose a precious hour of daylight.

Tonight Ed and I were taking my parents to dinner at Anthony's, while my uncle stayed home. He had complained of not feeling well, and as before, was having his dinner sent up. "I feel all gone," he said, which was a startling thing to hear if you'd not heard it before. So my husband and I had my mother and father to ourselves, although my mother could not shake her worry, and brought her cell phone along.

We had made our reservation in time for the sunset. Already my father was grieving that lost hour soon to come. "I hate to see it get dark so early," he said. He loved the light, and the early darkness oppressed him some way. We'd had a spectacular sunset, the sun laying golden ripples over the water before it disappeared behind the mountains off across the water. But the sun vanished too soon even now, and we all remarked on it. Still, it had been a beautiful sunset. And there was the water. We talked about all the good times we'd had, everybody in Hawaii when the kids were little and there were such promises to come. My uncle had always gone with us, and we talked about how much he too loved these trips.

Before the main course, my mother makes a check-in call. She says Henry sounds funny, disoriented.

"I fell," he says.

"Are you all right?"

"I don't know."

"Have you had your dinner?"

"I don't know."

"Where are you now?"

"In my chair."

So we leave our food on our plates and rush right home. We find him lying in bed, on his side. "Oh, it hurts," he says. My husband checks him over as best he can, moves his legs, feels around for pain.

"Do you want us to take you to the hospital?" I ask.

"Would I have to spend the night? I don't want to do that."

He knows how long it could take from waiting by the phone for word of my father's progress in the ER.

"It might be just a couple of hours," I say, none too convincingly.

"Oh I don't want to go. It doesn't hurt if I don't move. Maybe I'll be all right in the morning."

"Okay," we say, feeling the reprieve wash over us. "If you're sure. Because we could take you, you know."

I wasn't sure exactly how we'd get him to the car anyway without further injury if indeed something had really broken. We certainly knew how to call 911. But somehow it did not seem to be that sort of urgency. So we kissed him goodbye and went out the door. Looking back on it now we should have insisted, but we did not. And if we told the truth, we would say how secretly glad we were that he had refused us, that we had made our getaway and wouldn't have to spend half the night in the ER.

He hobbled around the apartment all of Monday, using my father's walker when he could. On Tuesday morning he fell again, this time in the bathroom. Now there was no question about calling 911, no question of where he was headed now. I was at the gym when the call came from my mother. As was my habit these days, I checked for messages first thing in the door, and rushed to the hospital in my gym clothes.

There he was, stretched out in the ER, a thin white blanket over his ancient pajamas.

"Oh, I'm so glad to see you," he says, taking my hand, as I materialize by his side. He looks up and there I am. I can see he's near tears.

"I'm so glad you're here," he says again. It's all true. I'm here, and will be here until the end. From now on I will be in charge, though I didn't know it at the time. My mother would pull back and devote all her energies to saving my father. I look down at my uncle's feet, sticking out from under the sheet. There are those awful gray socks he always wears with holes at the heel and one toe poking through. "Get those terrible socks off his feet," my mother had directed me just before I'd hung up the phone to dash to the hospital.

"Let's slip these off, Uncle Henry. They'll give you nice warm socks to wear. Aren't your feet cold?"

"I don't know," he says.

I kiss him and tell him everything's going to be all right, he's in the right place, they know what they're doing, he just has to be patient, which of course has never been his greatest strength. I wonder who he's terrorized already. But it doesn't matter. I'll patch things up so they wouldn't ignore him completely.

"I've just been lying here. They're not doing *anything* for me." I look at him lying on that bed and see my father and his anguish with the stroke in the ER. It's an echo that shatters my control.

"You know how it is in these places," I manage to say. "You just hold on. Everything's going to be okay."

I pull up a plastic chair and hold his hand. With the slightest move he cries out. They already know he's broken his back. *A significant break*, the doctor says. Of course, none of us will ever know if he had broken it in the first fall, the one he doesn't really remember, where he fell into his chair, put out his arms to break his fall and wrenched his back. I hoped selfishly, unforgivably, that he had not broken his back with that first fall, when we could have taken him to the hospital and saved him from the second fall that had broken his back for good. Now he'd had the fall that is so often the death knell of the elderly.

His doctor comes in, a nice man whom my uncle never took a liking to, not that there ever was a doctor he did like.

"Does this hurt?"

"I have no idea."

"Does it hurt when I do this?"

"I have no idea."

"Did you get dizzy before you fell?"

"I have no *idea*," he says, finally. "You're the doctor, you figure it out." I wonder what failure of language or thought he's masking.

A nurse comes in with a tall, lethal-looking glass of some kind of barium milkshake he is to drink. For some reason I cannot remember now and did not fathom at the time, they have to check something digestive.

My uncle looks suspiciously at the glass. "What's that for?"

"We need to take some digestive X-rays," she says carefully.

"Why would you do that? It's my *back* not my stomach!"

"Sir, it's what your doctor ordered."

"Where did you get your nursing degree? Did you have postgraduate training?"

She just stares at him, and hands me the glass. "Here." She's had enough already.

"Get him to take it in little sips. Try to get him to take it all, if you can." I could see the relief on her face as she turns on her heel and leaves the room.

"He's just scared," I say after her.

Apparently this is supposed to help them in sorting out which pains come from where, or at least that's what I told him. So I hold up his head with one arm and we get that ghastly stuff down, sip by sip, until he finally he says, "I can't take anymore."

I stay with him through the morning. When I return later in the afternoon, they have moved him out of the ER onto the telemetry floor. Why not orthopedics? "Where am I?" I ask at the nurses' station before I search out my uncle. "What's telemetry? He's broken his back. Why isn't my uncle on an orthopedic floor?"

"It's the floor where we can monitor the heart."

"But it's his back that's broken, not his heart."

"He's experiencing atrial fibrillation and an elevated heart rate, so he needs to be here." All right, so he has a fast-beating heart and now his old familiar syncopations. Well no wonder.

The next day the social worker tells me that after the hospital he will need an extended period of time in a convalescent center, i.e., rehab center, i.e., nursing home. She finds a place with an empty bed, which is our good fortune, I'm told, and my daughter and I check it out. There is a clown in the lobby of the Foss

Convalescence Home when we walk in. He hands us a balloon. It's a good omen, I say to myself, though I doubt if such things will cheer up my uncle. We visit the room that will be his, which he will share with a silent, gaunt man stretched out in the bed across the room. We look at the empty bed, the bed that will be his, shoved against the wall, in that windowless room with the yellow, faded light. The building is old, with long, linoleum hallways—a sad, wearing-down building with well-meaning but ineffectual attempts at cheer along the walls. And there's that rogue clown we'd seen in the lobby with the balloons. A sing-a-along is winding down in the recreation room. The pianist is pounding out "Strike Up the Band." A few of the residents clap in time to the music. It's all winding down. My daughter and I waltz down the hallway while several people in wheelchairs watch us, expressionless.

Send in the clowns, I say, whether you want them or not. Send in a thousand clowns every day of your life. I know in that instant that my uncle will never survive this place. Or they will never survive him.

Then it's evening and I come back down to the hospital to say goodbye. I'm headed off to a conference in Nebraska, to go to sessions, present a paper, see old friends, fly home. I will be gone four days. He's sleeping when I come into the room. I touch his arm to rouse him. He comes back from someplace far away. His face gleams with sweat. His arm feels hot.

Soon, an attendant comes in with a gurney. "We're taking him down to X-ray," he tells me.

"What for?" I want to know. That morning he'd been so tired I'd left him to sleep, and went off to finish packing, put the final touches on my paper, with the promise I'd come back in the evening to say goodbye. A nurse has come in and explains how yesterday he had choked and aspirated some fluid into his lungs. Now they're checking for pneumonia.

They maneuver him onto the gurney under protest. "I don't need a *chest* X-ray. You've got me confused with my *brother*. You people are always mixing up our files." And in truth they had. Not today, but too many times to count. Two identical men: *H Cunningham, d.o.b.: 6/9/13.*

But I have come too late for a proper goodbye. I tell him I'll just be gone a few days, and that I love him, and hope he's much better when I get back on Sunday. The diagnosis will be pneumonia. They will give him antibiotics and hope for the best. "Goodbye," I say, as they wheel him down the hall. He waves his arm vaguely. I wave back. Goodbye goodbye goodbye.

In forty-eight hours, while I wing my way to Nebraska then home again, he is propelled into a series of cascading events one after the other: aspiration pneumonia, a showering of tiny blood clots through his lungs and down his legs and feet, and gangrene has set in and his feet have turned black. Now a decision must be made whether to amputate his legs or let him die. But nothing will be decided until I can get there. He is moved from the telemetry floor—he'll need more than heart monitors now—down to the sixth floor, into the ICU. He is not expected to live. I do not go to sessions, I do not see friends, I do not give my paper.

I put on my sunglasses and hunker down in my cramped, airline seat. I look out the window at a cloudless sky and cry all the way home. When my husband meets me at the airport, he asks if I've caught a cold. But as soon as I land, the tears stop. My nose runs nonstop for the next three days. I think I must have a cold, but it is like no cold I have ever had before. But I have stopped the tears now for good. There will be no time for tears from now on. I ask my husband if everybody's still alive. I've been six hours out of phone contact. He just looks at me. We stand there for a minute, and I think my uncle has died. Then he pulls me into his arms and says, "Nobody's died."

"What?" I say. "What else has happened?"

"Annie, your father's in the hospital too." It's only what you would expect. The twins, Homer and Henry, would not be kept apart. My father had collapsed when they moved my uncle to the ICU, and even at that very moment was on the sixteenth floor of the same hospital where my uncle has been for a week now.

It's a sunny day I have flown into, but the light is even thinner than before. We go straight to the hospital. I see my uncle first. "Oh, you're back from your conference," he says as I come into the room, touch his arm. "How was it?" He has to remove the oxygen mask to say it. His face is puffy, and the oxygen mask has left deep creases in his skin.

"Fine," I say. I don't have to tell him anything else.

"Good," he says. "Good." He slips the mask back on and closes his eyes. I sit in the chair watching him sleep. His chest rises and falls with each breath. The heart rate monitor reads 110. There are other numbers that pulse and flash that I can't interpret. He has tubes and lines connected everywhere. The sheet is propped up at the end of the bed. I want to lift it and see his feet, to see if it's all really true, but cannot.

After a little while my uncle begins to tug at his gown and writhe a little. When the ICU nurse comes in, he tells her he has to go to the bathroom.

"Henry, you *can't* have to go to the bathroom, you have a *catheter*."

She leaves the room and he pulls the oxygen mask off his face and tells me he has to go to the bathroom so badly it hurts. I go back out and get the nurse.

"Something's wrong," I say.

She comes back in, clearly irritated. She checks the tubing, and sure enough the catheter is blocked and he can't empty his bladder. "Oh, I see what's wrong," she says, and clears the blockage. But she does not apologize for his discomfort. I want to yell at her. But in a moment she's gone and he's settled back into sleep. I know now I will have to watch over him every minute because I don't trust anyone to know what they're doing. I still have not seen my father. I still have not met Susan.

That night I do. "Where do you hurt, Henry?" Susan croons to him like a love song. She's the night ICU nurse who is an angel on this earth.

"Everywhere," he says. "I hurt *everywhere*." And in a choreography of such lightness and air, she shifts his pillow, smoothes out the blankets, adjusts his meds, and he can breathe again. Then she tucks him in for the long night, and he finds his way back to the comfort of sleep.

But his feet don't hurt. They don't feel a thing.

"They treat animals better than this," my mother says. She can't stand to visit him, see my uncle like this. She spends all her time sitting by my father's bed up on the sixteenth floor. Then I'm driving her home from the hospital back to the apartment at University House, where she lives now without the twins. It's a dress rehearsal for life without them, I'm thinking, but say nothing.

"This can't go on," she says.

"I know. I'll make it stop. I'll make this come to an end. The nurse already talked to me about it."

"Your father needs to say goodbye."

"Are you sure he'd want me to do this?"

"Oh, yes. He couldn't say it, though."

It's the next night and we're all assembled around my uncle's bed like a family portrait. We could be any family at the end of things, except for this strange, fierce current running between the man in the bed and the man in the wheel-chair who looks exactly like him. It's our visit to say goodbye and we all know it. My father knows it and I believe my uncle does too. My father had not thought he could do this, see his brother for the last time. But my mother said, "You'll be sorry forever if you don't. You can't ever call it back." We'd wheeled my father down to see him a couple of times these past days and they'd been wrenching enough. But though he is ill himself, he pulls the strength from somewhere, and says he would like to say goodbye to Henry after all. So we wheel him down from the sixteenth floor to the sixth floor, ten floors, to tell Henry goodbye.

My father's as close to the bed as his wheelchair will allow. He's sitting there with a white blanket over his thin white legs, another blanket over his shoulders. "I love you, Henry," my father says, taking his hand. Henry shakes his head, pulls at his oxygen mask. My husband lifts it carefully off Henry's face. My uncle tries to speak but cannot. He twists his head from side to side. Then he wails, for all that was, all that cannot be, for the end of things, the very end. But the cry makes no sound. Tears stream down his face. The pulse on the monitor jumps. My husband puts the mask back on Henry's face. We pat his arm, touch his forehead, his hands, touch his leg through the sheet. We do not go near the end of the bed. My father is crying. His shoulders slump. He can't take any more. He needs to go back to his room, lie down, shut his eyes. We leave the room with tears running unabashedly down our faces. Nobody says goodbye, but that's what it is.

Then my daughter and I slip back into the room and put three rose quartz crystals on my uncle's chest for the long night ahead. I knew then that I would lose them both. That my father would not survive my uncle's death, and I would enter that dark river of grief whose name I did not know.

As we leave I ask her about the crystals. "Tell me again about rose quartz."

"It's for healing the heart chakra."

Ah, for his syncopating, rushing heart. "Oh, good," I say. "His heart needs to stop racing."

"It's also for self-love."

"I hope so," I say. "He never had that." Maybe now he will. Maybe he'd have looked around the room last night and seen us gathered around his bed and known for sure how much he was loved, and finally love himself back.

I wondered what the morning shift nurse would think about those crystals. I never saw them again.

The next morning when I come into my uncle's room he knows exactly who I am, though he has to come back from a far, far place to meet me. I kiss him and tell him I love him, and he falls back into sleep or wherever it is he is going. I sit for a little while, watching his chest rise and fall as he pulls oxygen into his lungs with the help of everything they can give him short of intubation. I walk to the end of the bed and lift the sheet an inch or two and for the first time take a good hard look. For what's coming next I have to see for myself. His feet are charred. They have walked through the fire. Every impurity, every affront, insult, bitterness, regret, purified by this fire spreading even now up his legs. But no pain. No pain at all. That's why I know this is the necessary fire.

Then I leave him without looking back and go down the hall into the family conference room to meet with his doctors and nurses and the social worker, to decide what should be done, but there is only one thing to be done, and right now I'm the only one who can do it, for I am the only family member here. It's first thing in the morning, and my mother is still at home, and of course my father is ten floors up, and my husband is stuck in a traffic jam miles away. We are going to spare the children this final scene.

They call him a "sundowner" now, a word that distances him already, and tells exactly where he's going. The doctor counts the ways Uncle Henry's life is, for all practical purposes, over. Back broken in two places. Months of rehab ahead. Aspiration pneumonia. Blood clots. Gangrene. The doctor goes on, but I can only think of his blackened, charred feet, and that the only thing that will save him now, though he can't be saved, is the double amputation they're recommending, which is too obscene even to think about.

Sitting around this conference table I think of him right there with us, and wonder what his vote would be, but he can't tell us now, so the four of us vote to remove the oxygen mask, stop pushing the blood pressure meds, and see what happens, though I'm the only one with the real vote. It may not even happen right away. It could take hours or even days, though I can't imagine it.

But don't worry, they tell me, "we'll just move him out of ICU up to the sixteenth floor."

"The sixteenth floor!" I say. "He can't be on the 16th floor. His brother's up there." The sixteenth floor was a place to make you well, not a place for you to die. My father is no sundowner, I want to scream. Then a chilling thought comes to me. His *identical twin* brother is on the sixteenth floor. I'd seen my father's name on the patient reader board above the nurses' station all week: *H Cunningham, 6/9/13*. I'm a little crazy by then and have to work to suppress a laugh.

"So. How does this work exactly?" I ask. "The patient board has *two H Cunningham*s with *6/9/13* birthdays. Two patients who look exactly alike even now, and you're going to keep all this straight? They've had their medical records mixed up before." I look out with furious eyes.

"Oh," they say, "we hadn't thought of that."

"My father can't have his brother down the hall," I say more quietly now, but unyieldingly. "He's already said goodbye."

But it takes only minutes before he starts to go. All they have done is remove his oxygen mask. I'm in the hall talking to Father Bill, the ICU priest who had come by yesterday. "Why do you work here? How can you stand it?"

And he says, "Oh, but this is a luminous place. It shimmers, if only you can see it. There's a thin membrane separating the physical and the spiritual. We should walk with one foot in each place always. This place reminds me to do that. It's a thin place."

I look up and there is Susan rushing down the hall to me. "He's going."

Now that the oxygen mask is gone, I can see my uncle's face. His eyes are open. I tell him how much I love him, kiss his forehead, stroke his arm. He doesn't mind it now. Yesterday, he had edged his arm away from me. I did not understand this avoidance of touch. He's going to another place now and doesn't want to be called back. But I didn't know it then and so I kept touching him anyway. Finally I said, "Do you want me to touch you?" No, my uncle had told me. No.

Now his breathing changes. Two little puffs of breath, then a long, breathless silence that stretches out between one world and another until he catches it up again and pulls himself back into this life. He's emptying the body of air. But there is no gasping, no death agony, as I'd been warned, just little puffs of air, little commas of breath, the sweet, soft sound of the spirit going someplace else. His eyes are open. The light has not gone out. All the times I had left him, and gone home to eat or sleep, to take up the threads of my life as best I could, and I thought please let go, please let this all be over, please just slip away softly into the night. Now I am grateful to be here and think how easily I might not have been.

"What's happening to him?" I ask Susan. She explains how systems are shutting down, one after the other.

"What is happening to his spirit?" I ask Father Bill.

"He's becoming pure spirit now, what he was and always will be. He's going to it now. Everything else is falling away."

His chest is quiet now, and the light has gone from his eyes though they are still open. "We can give him something to close them," Susan says. Tears run down her face. I am grateful for her tears because right then she is everybody who loves him who is not here. And then as if on cue, his eyes close slowly, sweetly as in a dream, because that's exactly where he's going. His face is smooth as he eases into death. He's as beautiful to me now as ever. All the outrages and grievances of his life have been washed away with his suffering.

The fog has burned off, and I see the cold true light of October above the Seattle skyline as I wait to take the elevator for the last time from the ICU floor to the sixteenth floor, where my father is. I'd been taking that elevator between those two floors for days now. For a moment I see what Father Bill meant about this place, which suddenly I do not want to leave. I want to go back down the hall and sit in one of the little family rooms for a while. I do not want to see my father. I do not want to give him the news.

My uncle was born first. My father, the unbreathing one, was born second, and laid in a little basket they put by the stove, so the doctor could concentrate on the only twin he thought could be saved. But of course my father lived, or I would not be here telling this story. My uncle always joked that his lifelong foot trouble came from having to carry my father around in the womb all those months. But all through their lives they took turns carrying each other, and that is why the story of one is always the story of the other. To see your face forever looking back at you, hear your voice in the air, you who are also me, my secret sharer, my double, to be forever one half of a whole, then one gone from the other forever. How to unravel this tangling of lives no stretch of years or miles could untie? My father and uncle lived in a thin place all their lives, each with a foot in the world of the other, with but a scrim of separation between them.

My uncle had bought a thousand pairs of shoes in his life, but those last years wore only one. They were worn down at the heel such that his feet hardly stayed in them. The year before he died he bought a pair of Scandinavian walking shoes for three hundred dollars, which he never wore, which stayed in their box in his closet until his birthday six months later, when I wrapped them up as a birthday present. He never knew the difference. "Thank you," he said, but they stayed in the box.

It was the same with the socks. Those same gray socks with the holes I had slipped off him in the ER. They were his favorite brand, which had been discontinued years ago. So he wore the same couple of pairs full of holes over and over, though after he died and we went through his drawers, we found dozens of brand-new pairs saved for a future that would never come. We buried him in his Scandinavian walking shoes, his see-through yellow shirt, his brown pants, his brown plaid jacket.

A few weeks after his death, he comes to me in a dream. He's wearing his burial clothes. He smiles at me and I say, "Oh, I know you're dead, but I'm so glad to see you." But it's as close to him as I could get. I was too busy getting my father set up in the "rehab" facility, i.e., *nursing home*, we'd had to transfer him to when he became too well to stay in the hospital and too sick to go home.

When my father was well enough, we held a memorial service for my uncle at University House. When it came time for him to speak, my father tried to give a little revival sermon, much to the mortification of my mother. He thought if he told how his brother had finally come to God, he might save some souls in the audience, perhaps even us. Maybe if we all heard the story of my uncle coming to God, we would come to God too. But he stopped after the first couple of sentences and just sat in his wheelchair and cried. He wiped his eyes, and my husband wheeled him back to his place in the audience.

I was too busy keeping my father in this life for signs from the other side. "Henry keeps calling me. He says to come on up," my father tells me. "He says it's time. I can't just ignore it." Then he adds, "Don't tell your mother."

No. Nothing like that. I didn't even think to look for signs or symbols. But my father saw it and so did my daughter. She walked in that thin place I could not find. And in that thin place, my uncle came to her. My daughter had asked my uncle for a sign. "Tell me that you're there," she'd said. "Tell me that you're somewhere."

The next day my daughter is sitting beside my father. He's all stretched out in his "rehab bed" as they're calling it, until he gets back on his feet and can go home. He's wearing his khaki Dockers and his tan sports shoes, his beige sweater. He's weeping from such a deep place it frightens her. She leans over and hugs him. Then she's asked to leave the room while they help him to the bathroom. When she comes back in the room, he's holding something in his hand.

"It's Henry's watch!" he says in astonishment. "I found it in my pocket. I don't know how it got here. Here, Courty, you take it. You keep it safe." And so she does. No one can remember or account for how my uncle's watch got into my father's pocket, or how he happened to find it just then. Of course there is a logical explanation somewhere, yet the heart rejects logic for a deeper truth.

So it's truth I'm after when I go through my uncle's things. I feel like a voyeur, and yet that is what families do after the end of things. Better to burn everything before you go. Among his possessions after his death, and the single thing I have kept for myself, is a Tampa Nugget cigar box, his boyhood box of precious things he'd kept all his life. Would this box explain my uncle to me? Or would it call forth more mysteries yet, and only increase the poignancy of his life, which insisted itself so strongly on our own?

He'd written his initials, *HWC*, on all sides of that Tampa Nugget cigar box, and across the top he'd written his name, *Henry Wayne Cunningham*, as if practicing his adult signature, as kids do, imprinting his name upon the world. But my Uncle Henry wasn't born *Henry* at all, nor was he Henry when he was that little boy, practicing his name. His given name was Wayne Emerson Cunningham. And when he was twelve, he said he didn't want to be called "little Wayne" anymore. He was the "smaller" of the twins, though not by any measure you'd notice. Still, he didn't want any name that defined him in comparison to his brother. He wanted to be called *Henry* from now on, after his favorite uncle. And when he was an adult he officially changed his name. On that Tampa Nugget cigar box, my uncle was beginning a transformation that would take him farther from my father and also bring him closer. James Gatz to Jay Gatsby. Wayne Emerson to Henry Wayne.

All kids go through that phase of wanting to change their name. As a child I lamented my plain and unadorned first name that did not even have an elegant "e" on the end, which I had always wanted to give myself but never did. Somehow, like it or not, I would be *Ann* to the world and to myself. Yet here was my uncle. He wasn't a famous movie star who'd been forced to shed his clunky given name for a glamorous studio one. He wasn't a John Wayne, whose first name was Marion, or a Cary Grant, who was born Archibald Leach. He was just little *Wayne*, who changed his name to *Henry*, giving my father and my uncle virtually the same set of initials—*HFC* and *HWC*, and two *H Cunninghams, d.o.b.: 6/9/13* in hospitals and doctor's offices and elsewhere, for the rest of their lives. *Homer and Henry*, the twins, now and forever.

It was like this: we're all in Hawaii, on a beach walk, and one of the twins makes that terrifying turn to find the other gone. And there it is, like a refrain all through their lives: Where's Henry? Where's Homer? Are you all right, Homer?

Are you all right, Henry? Are you there? Just so you're there. Was my uncle's name change a way of turning toward my father or away? Ah, but we're all unknowable in the end, to others and to ourselves.

In that box I found a set of typed 3 x 5 cards with the text of a debate or speech on the merits of grocery chains, envelopes addressed to his mother and father but no letters, an envelope full of stamps, graphite rocks wrapped in waxed paper, both his parents' watches, a family portrait, an art school application, a wedding ring.

I make my astonished way through these things one by one. And what to make of those fourteen typed index cards, kept all these years? Had it won some contest or debate? Did he win a trophy? Was his name in the paper? The speech is addressed to "Mr. Chairman and Friends" and concludes:

> *Yet the chains in no way harm our economic structure but rather put business on a firmer basis. It is a natural development of modern business and not some huge monster who has just recently come to life. We have no objection to the independent merchant. Let the independents continue to serve the people as they always have...There is really no quarrel between them. They do not hinder each other. They have their respective places.*

When the appearance of the chain stores threatened a whole way of life, or so it seemed, my uncle had come down on the side of progress. But to keep those cards all these years, tucked into that cigar box with his parents' watches, I wondered what dreams hoped for, or what dreams lost, they truly held. What sense of himself was resurrected when he looked at them? What victory or defeat did they mean? How did they tell him who he was?

And the watches.

My grandfather's watch from Alfreda was simply inscribed: *James from*

Alfreda, Nov 11, 1910, a birthday present seven months before their marriage, his birthday the same as my husband's. And inside the watch her picture looking out at him properly, seriously, as was the custom. But her promise never to smile again haunts that picture. I look again at her somber face and try to see behind the set expression. And there it is, a certain resignation or defiance behind the eyes, as if to prove she wasn't kidding. I had never thought of Alfreda as my grandmother. I could see nothing of myself in her face. The only time we were ever linked was in her obituary, which my uncle had saved all these years, and which I read for the first time going through that box. There I was, ten days old, her first and only grandchild, a granddaughter named *Ann*, whom she would never see.

And a family portrait: A mother and father and two little boys, one on each lap, dated February 23, 1918. The Great War. The year of the great flu pandemic. My father and uncle are five years old. My grandfather is looking directly into the camera. In fact, he's smiling into it, and it's a lovely smile. His eyes are sharp and bright as though the world is a fine place and there is everything to look forward to, as though terrible things have not happened, that this is a family unscathed by disease or war. He's holding my father on his lap, who's smiling too. Alfreda is looking off to the right of the camera. Her unsmiling face matches my uncle's, who's looking in the same direction.

But how do I know this, when there is no one now to ask to be sure? And no writing on the back of the photograph to identify who is who. Why does this seem so important? Oh, it's either Homer or Henry. It's either one or the other, after all. I could say that my father tended to smile in pictures and my uncle did not; that from a certain angle and in just the right light, my father's face seemed a little broader, his eyes a little wider. They are dressed identically in all the family photos I can find: little sailor suits, jackets and knickers, beanies and caps, sitting or standing on little wooden horses, swings, wheelbarrows, chairs. Even in their infant pictures, four months old, and dressed in their white, baptismal gowns, I can tell who's who. Both are on the verge of laughter at someone off camera who's caught their eye and beckoned those smiles—maybe the photographer's assistant or their mother or father. I imagine this matter of photographs drives to the core of the divided heart of any identical twin. When so much of one's identity comes from this pairing, how the soul must long for separation, even as that separation is one's greatest fear. Ah, the family portrait. Images and shadows of the family unit from which all else derives, despite our best intentions and our deepest desires.

But to me, the most poignant item in that box was a certificate of "scholarship" to something called the *North American School of Drawing* my uncle had supposedly won by submitting a drawing of the profile of a balding, large-nosed man, with a half-smile and a cigar. It would hardly have been a natural subject for a boy of thirteen, living in a parsonage in Lakeland, Florida. I had seen such a thing in a magazine when I was a child. DRAW ME, it said, and so he did. The letter was addressed to Mr. Henry Cunningham, offering the possibility of fame and fortune in commercial drawing:

> *It is not unusual to hear of men and women residing in remote country districts making good incomes from the sale of their drawings done in their spare time.*

And in a separate typed "Memo":

> *There is a certain freedom in your work which is very pleasing and which is not usually found in a beginner's drawing.*

He'd have waited upon the mail week after week for this letter from Buffalo, New York, all the way to 701 Peachtree Street, Lakeland, Florida. Then here it was at last. I imagined a factory full of women typing away and sending out these letters to wistful teenage boys. Of course the "scholarship" meant that he would only have to pay $47.50 instead of the regular $100 for a year's instruction, to be paid as five dollars down and five dollars a month until the sum was paid in full.

But "*If you are under 21 years of age this Agreement must be signed by your Parent or Guardian.*" All these years, he had kept this application for the scholarship he had won, never filled out, never sent in. I wonder now if my uncle had ever shown his parents this drawing of a man smoking a cigar. Drinking and smoking and dancing and gambling and just about everything else was forbidden in their religion. A man with a cigar wasn't *art*. This wasn't a *real* scholarship. It was just a hoax. He hadn't won anything at all. Yet my uncle had kept all of it—the critique saying he had "talent," the letter describing the program of study that held such promise of success, and the drawing itself. A boyhood dream counts for something in the final tallying up of one's life—what might have been and never was.

But then, oh then, at the very bottom of the box, under everything—a *ring*. Underneath the papers and note cards and clippings there was a man's 14 K gold wedding ring. His parents never wore rings. They were considered ornamentation, and against their Free Methodist religion. A watch was practical. A ring was an adornment. Since my uncle had never married, whose ring could this have been? I had never seen my uncle wear such a ring. I had never seen him wear any ring at all. Even in his father's second marriage, J.B. would have worn no ring. And even if he had, Lillian would have kept it, not my uncle. Had the ring been given to him by the woman he had once loved and who had left him? "I shall never marry," my uncle had said. A pronouncement that closed down his life, and determined all that was to come, just like Alfreda's promise never to smile again.

I take the ring to a jeweler to be polished up, which is only partly successful. Then I take it in to my mother's and compare it to my father's wedding ring. I expected if not an exact match, a close one, but there is no such thing. It's so large my father's ring slips right through it. I had thought my uncle might have worn it to lend a little respectability to his hotel visits all those Saturday nights in Detroit. This biggest clue of all I could not read. As a boy had he picked it up off the street and carried it in his pocket, then put it for safekeeping in his little Tampa Nugget cigar box? Why a wedding ring saved with other precious things by a man who vowed he would never marry?

I am a genuine intruder now. These things my uncle would never have wished us to know. Yet how precious they are to me, even in all their contradiction. These little things are artifacts now. Relics. Sacred objects, signposts, markers along the way. I look again at my uncle's little box. It's so small and it makes me so sad. *Rosebud, Rosebud.*

"Your mother never loved you. That's why you're the way you are," the psychiatrist had said. Imagine hearing that. Imagine a professional saying that to someone already despairing over his damaged life. Alfreda had died, and there was no asking her if that shrink was right after all. "Why didn't you love me? Why did you love my brother more than you loved me?" The twins had not shared the watches. I can hear my father saying, "Go ahead, Henry, you take it," when their mother died. And then when their father died, saying it again. I can see my uncle, forging his own identity against the miraculous goodness of my father, and my uncle's sense of deprivation and want everywhere he turned. There was no list of my uncle's hundred lovers, not anywhere, not that we ever found.

My father had no such box. My father had such plenitude, there was no need to carry talismans from an earlier life wherever he went. But I do have my father's historical photographs, newspaper articles about him, his class notes, a few sermon notes. And I have the one and only book he wrote: *The Presidents' Last Years*, typed by my mother and edited by me, our single collaboration, if that does not give my own part too much importance. Yet what I have of him goes far deeper than a childhood box. I do not have to peel the layers away to find my father.

Yet if my father had had a box of unspent dreams, it might have held ribbons and medals for running. My father loved to run and always won every race with his brother, and most of the other boys. He wanted to join the high school track team when they lived in Spring Arbor, but was forbidden this by his father. It was his great adolescent sorrow, as school dances had been mine. But at Greenville College he played basketball and then went on as a faculty member to coach the men's basketball team for several years, until my mother made him quit because he got so worked up it was giving him an ulcer. But later he became Greenville College's first athletic director, in addition to his position as professor of history. The year after his stroke, the college named him to the Athletic Hall of Fame, and I wondered about the irony of it and if he felt it too. They sent him a plaque, which he kept on the end table by his chair. He could go down the river of memory that held his body in its fullness, mitigating for a time the walker and the wheelchair.

My father and I both loved sports, and we shared that world, especially during my junior high years. By then we'd been living in Spokane for several years, and since my father was on the faculty at Whitworth College, we had the use of the college gym, which we used on weekends to practice free throws. I could almost always beat him in H-O-R-S-E, never thinking, of course, that he might have set it up that way. He'd coach me on my layups and help me with my hook shot, which I thought was the most elegant move in basketball, with your arm in a graceful, balletic arch over your head as the ball just floats off the tip of your fingers.

There are two memories I would tuck away in a little secret box if I had had one. The first is a basketball game against Deer Park, our crosstown rivals, played on February 2, on my fourteenth birthday. My team is one point behind, with forty-five seconds to go in the game, when somebody fouls me going in for a layup, and I get two free throws. I make them both. We win by one, and it's the best birthday I ever had.

The second comes a year later, in the spring of the ninth grade. My father takes me to the Whitworth College track in the early evenings to help me practice my broad jump, in preparation for the Eastern Washington Junior Olympics, which I had earlier qualified for. I win a silver medal in those Junior Olympics.

"How did it go?" my father says, as I bound off the bus and slide into the car.

I smile and hold up my silver medal, but don't say a thing, because I haven't really won second place after all. I've tied for it. He's so proud of me when I show him my silver medal that I can't diminish his pride in me by even the fraction of an inch I would have had to leap to win it free and clear. But somehow over the years I lost that medal, never having made a place to keep such things safe from the chaos of my growing up. I have no such box of treasures. I was more like my father than my uncle, with little need for saving totems and icons from my past. Maybe we had less to prove to ourselves than my uncle did.

My father and I spent many of my junior high summer evenings out on the patio of the first real house we ever had, that little two-bedroom house in Spokane where my grandparents also lived, before my grandfather died, the house that could accommodate a dog at last. My father and I would sit out on cool summer nights, listening to the Spokane Indians baseball games on the radio, keeping box scores to the sound of the crickets and the thump of the baseball in the mitt and crack of the ball on the bat. I was stretched out on a chaise lounge with my dachshund, Heidi, snuggled up beside me, my clipboard propped against my legs. Earlier that afternoon I'd been practicing my swing out in the backyard and accidentally clipped Heidi in the head. She ran in circles, shrieking. It was the most terrible sound I had ever heard. Then she stopped and just stood there looking blankly, and lay down and shut her eyes. I had killed her. I started to scream. My very own dog at last, whom I loved even more than I loved my parents. But finally she got up, shook her head, and licked my hand. It's all right, she said, but don't do that again. I sat on the lawn hugging her for a long time. In that moment, I realized how quickly things could change, how fragile our hold on this earth. What terrible things a person could do without even trying.

But here we were, tucked under the awning in that warm summer air. Those summer nights seemed to have a completeness and magic all their own. The bamboo grown up around the patio made it into a little green bower of safety, and I had the feeling that we would all live forever. I had not killed my dog after all. She was snuggled up beside me, with no such thing as life lived in fast-forward, seven years at a time.

I loved the Dodgers too, as the Spokane Indians were a farm club for the Dodgers, and we'd listen to those games as well. I wasn't trying to be my father's son. I was always and only myself. Yet there were things a daughter couldn't ask her father. It was the night the Dodgers were playing the Yankees. The sportscaster kept talking about a Yankee right fielder named Penis Slaughter. I jumped the first time I heard his name shouted out, and listened closely every time he was at bat or fielded a ball to see if that's what I had really heard. His first name couldn't *really* be Penis. How could anyone name their kid something like that? Of course his name was *Enos*, but I had never heard that name before and didn't even know there was such a name. But it embarrassed me to be hearing what sounded like *Penis* over the radio in my father's presence, so I didn't laugh, as I would have with my seventh-grade friends, or ask my father if that could possibly be his name. Sex, like death, was years away from my thirteen-year-old mind. I was in no hurry to grow up. I wanted everything to stay like this forever.

My father was too shy to take any real part in my sex education, leaving it in the hands of my capable guidance counselor–mother. He had only two things to impart. The first involved the dangers of school dances, of course, and the second was whatever he meant when he asked me "You know how boys can take advantage of girls, don't you?"

"Sure," I said, having absolutely no idea what he meant. But the way he framed the question made it easy to say what he wanted so to hear.

"Oh, *good*," he said. Even I could tell how relieved he was that he would not have to explain such things, that somehow this was my mother's job.

Sometimes I think my father felt excluded when my mother and I went off for a day of shopping and lunch or in the summertime when we went to the river to float in our inner tubes, then lie on the beach in the sun. Basketball, volleyball, softball, track. It was a way he could know he and I were special too.

It's my junior year of college and Vietnam has exploded all around us. Ed has a 2A draft status, an education deferment, but it's not going to last forever. He's from a rural draft district and they're hard-pressed to fill their quota. If there is only to be now, if now is the only future we're ever going to have, why not get married and have what family we can? It's sooner than either of my parents expected, but we don't care.

Soon enough my future husband's on his way downstairs, where my father is waiting for him in the rec room, where he will declare his intentions. My mother had told me it would be a courtesy for him to ask my father for my hand in marriage, even though nothing is going to stop us. Ed has never heard of such a thing. That was okay. He'd do whatever he needed to. My mother and I are in the kitchen, waiting it out. Of course, this has all been set up in advance, preceded by a dinner out with just the four of us. But Ed's nervous and wants this part to be over.

He sits down across from my father at the card table my father has set up. It looks like it's going to be an interrogation.

"Well, son, there's one thing you have to do if you're going to become a member of this family," my father tells him first thing.

Ed has no idea what this thing could be. Of course he's willing to do just about anything. And how bad could it be? But he was from a Catholic family and I was Presbyterian, which had already caused both sets of parents some distress. The parish priest had told his parents it would be a sin to attend our marriage, since it would be a Protestant wedding. No wonder Ed was uneasy. Maybe

Protestants had their own strange rules. Maybe he would have to convert. Become Presbyterian in front of a large group of people. Recite the Apostles' Creed.

"Now this is the deal," my father says, "and there's no way around it."

"Okay," Ed says with a gulp.

"You've got to learn to play golf."

"Golf?" he says. "I can do that."

Now both of them are smiling, and my father shakes his hand. "Welcome to the family."

At this time my husband was going to the University of Washington on a football scholarship, but in the summer he had already begun to learn to golf, and like my father, soon loved it passionately, as golfers do, loved it almost as much as he loved fishing for salmon. It was a way they could be together. It was a language they could share. And then in his career, my husband, like my father, became an athletic director too. So sports became a metaphor between them for the affection they held for each other but could not say out loud. I'm not sure my father ever knew how much my husband loved him, though my husband felt my father's love always.

My father was always surprised when a former student remembered him and greeted him with great warmth. He loved easily, unconditionally, and was so forgiving of human frailties that people always loved him back extravagantly. Yet he was sometimes a little surprised at this. I never saw it, but once or twice my mother called from Spokane to tell me my father felt a little down. Could I call him just to chat? "He feels sad, sometimes," she said. "Sometimes he feels he's not good enough." Because in his deepest heart, my father, like his brother, worried that he was not loved either. What my uncle felt for sure, my father only feared occasionally. Maybe deep down something had been withheld from him also. He was always working hard to be loved. He wanted so earnestly to be funny that sometimes his jokes missed the mark with his grandchildren, and offended their growing social sensibility.

Yet Henry blamed my father for a favoritism that may or may not have been. "You got the best bike," he said to my father when they were in their late seventies, while my mother sat the silent listener, as they did their old two-step around the subject of their childhood. A tangling of love even in the womb, that pull and tug between them across the years and miles. Maybe their parents had played them against each other, taking unforgiving turns with their affections. Maybe there was not enough love to go around. And Alfreda—maybe she hadn't enough left over to give to these little boys, always at the same stage of life. Maybe they chose their parts to show their difference. How they must have wanted to be loved as a single, solitary self and not half of a whole.

Bessie Burton

Bessie Burton was the first thing we saw when we came through those sliding doors into that dark lobby, my father on the gurney from the ambulance that had brought him from the hospital for this brief "rehab" stay, till he could get on his feet. In her lofty portrait on the far wall, Bessie sat looking out over that dark lobby, smiling so calmly, so benignly, you'd never know what horrors she watched over. She was the wealthy grandmother you never had, her gray hair in a knot on top of her aristocratic head, as the artist had rendered her in oils for all eternity. The lace collar on her paisley V-necked dress, the ample bosom, the hands folded in her lap, the works. You could almost hear her say it: Fear not. Come unto me all ye who labor and are heavy laden and I will give you rest.

I had no idea who she was.

Yesterday my father was in the hospital trying to gain back enough strength to walk down that sixteenth-floor hall for the required one hundred feet, which it turned out he could not do, when suddenly, precipitously, or so it seemed, they released him from the hospital. Today I'm at school just before getting ready to dash off to class when the social worker calls me to say they're releasing my father that afternoon, where did I want him to go? Medicare would not pay for a single extra hour. I would have to find a nursing home that would accept him. She said I should do some Internet research and pick a place.

"Now?" I say.

Yes, now. Are you deaf? "He has to be released by two this afternoon, and he's got to go somewhere."

I know nothing of nursing homes. But I finally manage to find a web site in between classes, though I can tell nothing from it. Everyplace has black marks for something: food kept unsafe, patient–nursing staff ratio, patients in restraints, medication errors. There is no end of things to send him into harm's way. But the social worker and I finally settle on Bessie Burton, because of its reputation as a good rehab facility, and more to the point, the bed that has just become available. At that time my father's not yet considered a *longtimer*, so all we want is a place that will take him right now, a place that can be endured for the sake of what the social worker has called good physical therapy.

My mother and I take the transport elevator up with my father's gurney to the second floor, and the medics maneuver the gurney down the hall and into what will be his room for the duration. A yellowy light, as if from an old lamp-shade, hangs over everything like ancient dust, as ancient as the picture of Bessie Burton herself. It's as depressing a place as the one we had looked at for my uncle, only there was no clown with a thousand balloons, no "Strike Up the Band."

They stick my father into a tiny bed in the corner, an ancient bed, with a hand crank, to raise and lower the head of the bed, which means he can't change his position himself, but must wait until someone comes to crank him up or crank him down. The bed is so low it's impossible for him to get in or out of it on his own. This bed seems of another century, like the building itself. My father is pinioned to it. The room has no television bolted to the wall or anywhere. The residents can bring in their own, but where could we put it? My father's side of the room is a cubicle. The only place possible is in a tiny walk-way between the wall and the bed. We'll bring my uncle's TV and his little TV stand and see what happens.

What else can he do to pass the hours in that bed but watch TV? He can't read anymore, and we can't be there every hour of every day. And how my father had come to love television. How he loved to change channels. It's the only way he can go anywhere on his own. But lying in that narrow bed wedged against the wall, shoved in a corner like that, he seems diminished, like he had lost a great deal of weight. Well, he has no brother now. Half of him has fallen away.

My father's roommate is named Max. His daughter comes every evening and complains about how much work she has to do at home, how much time all these visits are taking. Occasionally a child, bored out of his mind, accompanies her, with no seeming connection to the man in the bed, and now and then a husband comes along. Max had been a professor of fisheries at the University of Washington. Two college professors for roommates. Maybe they can strike up a friendship. Talk about history and fish. Life in academia. Politics. Economics. But the only thing Max ever says to my father is to shout at him to turn off his television.

Max is a big man. He commands two-thirds of the room space, which includes a wall of windows and a ledge with plants and flowers and a big television in the corner, which is turned up loud enough to hear it in the hall. The light from those windows is blocked most of the time by the curtain that is often drawn between them. And even without that curtain, the light from those windows never quite reaches my father's bed, jammed as it is against the wall. Max has a high, modern bed with buttons to push for going up and going down. Maybe that's why he seems so much bigger than my father. He sits in that bed like a king on a throne.

Max continues to complain about my father's TV. He calls a nurse to order my father to turn his television off—not down, but *off*. And my father just slides more deeply into himself, and does not protest or cry out to say, *But I'm here too*. I have as much right to watch television as you do. Before, he would have stood up for himself. And he would have loved to tell the story, punching up the words in all the right places. It's an aching testimony to the way he's shrinking before my very eyes, the way he is diminished, even to himself. In fact, he never watches his TV again, though we buy him earphones so he could do so without setting off Max. But by now he has forgotten how to use the controls, has forgotten how to put on the earphones, and then he loses interest in watching anything altogether.

I took a strange liking to Max despite his imperious ways with my quiet father. I should have hated him. In part, I guess I did. But I saw something gentle in him also, despite his bluster. He was a big man. A turtle on its back. What exactly his diagnosis was we never learned. They had to bring in a lift just to get him in and out of bed—a contraption that was sort of a scaffold, a metal hangman's platform with a sling, instead of a noose. Later, they would use one of these for my father, when two aides, one on each side, could not get him up out of bed either.

"Hello, Max," I'd say, hoping it would help him be nicer to my father. All Max ever managed was a mumbled hello back. Then one day he looked me up and down. "You're pretty thin," he said, flirting with me in a bald, unpracticed way. I wondered if he'd been a ladies' man. I wondered who he had been before he wound up on his back like that. There was no wife. Only that much-put-upon daughter, a grandchild, perhaps a former student or two.

"You're pretty thin," he says again.

"Well, I guess so," I say and smile back. You be nice to him. You be nice to my father.

"I can't sleep," my father complains. "That man across the hall makes too much noise." It was disconcerting, even by day, to hear those moans above the clatter and thrum of the halls. We call him The Wailer. It isn't a shout or a cry he makes, but a long unending moan. He isn't calling out for anything or anyone. It's just a long, loud wail beyond significance. I try to imagine that sound in the middle of the night as you lie there trying to find sleep, and what dark place that sound would take you to. Maybe it's a way of not going gently into the night that had already tucked you in for good. Ah, Bessie Burton. Her real work was this after all. Don't be suckered in by that thin smile of hers, those cool, imperious eyes.

And then one evening the lights were turned out in that poor man's room, except for a tiny bed light, or maybe a candle. A man was sitting beside the bed of The Wailer, who made no sound now. He was reading something out loud to him, perhaps a Bible. From across the hall it wasn't even a whisper. You only knew that man was reading out loud by the way his lips moved. He was there all evening, maybe all night. And the next day The Wailer was gone.

"Last night at dinner, your father choked," Marie, another patient, tells me. "People with strokes often have trouble swallowing. You should get him to a speech therapist." She'd called me over and I'd come and sat in a chair beside her. She had dark, shining eyes, short-cropped gray hair, and two purple casts—one on her left arm and one on her right leg. A nasty fall and now here she was, wheelchair-bound and in a nursing home. You couldn't walk on crutches or a walker with only one good leg and one good arm. She lived alone and had no one to help her get around. So she found herself at Bessie Burton along with others who could not get themselves up or down.

She got around by pushing one wheel with the good arm and scooting herself with her good leg. Nobody was going to have to wheel *her* around. It was impossible to tell how old she was. She held all the life you'd ever need in those dark, flashing eyes. By then she'd made a whole network of friends to whom she seemed to be a sort of den mother or camp counselor. Now here she was, looking after us too. She had seen the future and she had seen the past.

As it turned out, the speech therapy got lost in the shuffle of the next days and my father's precipitous release, though we picked the therapy up later, sometime after he'd come home to University House, when a speech therapist came to the apartment to assess his swallowing. Swallowing had provided the fatal moment for my uncle. After Uncle Henry had aspirated into his lungs, he could not recover. And so we were all thinking of that, and that first dinner at University House when my father almost died from swallowing wrong. I did not know it then, but we were in far country now. And this difficulty in swallowing was one of the landmarks we failed to read.

From the speech therapist we learned that we'd been doing everything wrong. Very hot and very cold liquids were best. These wake up the sleepy nerves in the mouth and throat, get the esophagus ready for whatever is coming down the pipe. Cool or tepid things can slide right down unnoticed, into the lungs. We'd had enough of that. Liquids through a straw are dangerous, also. Maybe that's what had happened to my uncle. Maybe he'd tried to drink from a straw. Then why did everybody in a hospital get a straw with their drink? That was easy. So they wouldn't dump their drink down their front and need a bed change.

Now as days followed days at Bessie Burton, my father grew thinner, slighter. He said little. He sank deeply into depression, and I knew he could only be saved by getting him out of there as soon as possible. The kids took turns visiting him, and though he loved it, loved just looking at them or touching their hands, he would grow quiet a few minutes into the visit, and often fall asleep. One night my son Chris wheeled him into the little visitors' room to watch the World Series. This way they wouldn't bother Max and risk an outburst. The only baseball game my father ever saw Chris play was the only time he ever hit a triple. They talked about that, sitting in the little TV alcove, watching the Series. I'd said to Chris that afternoon, "It will be the last time this can ever be. You remember this." And so he did, in this poem:

> We are having a good talk now over the baseball game
> the very last time we were feeling this good both at the same time
> a twinkle in that wink
> then planet leaving half-last breath.

Ninety Days

T hen one day my father is suddenly released from the nursing home. Now my mother is on her own with him. It's shocking, this expulsion. She calls me at work. "They're releasing your father tomorrow," she says in a panic. As much as they hated that place, it was worse to be going home. "There has to be some mistake," I say when I call Bessie Burton. But it was no mistake. As before, Medicare has called the shots. He'd gone as far as he could go in physical therapy. He was as rehabilitated as he would ever be. So it was an expulsion after all. My mother would be alone with him now. It should have been cause for celebration, except for the loss that had made it possible. Yet they'd talked of it, how they had some good years left. My mother told me how much he missed touching her, and loving her in the old way.

So my husband and I gather up his things—his TV, his radio, my mother's picture, his pajamas, his extra clothes—and help him into the front seat of our van and head home. Goodbye Max. Goodbye Bessie Burton. We had decorated the apartment at University House with *Welcome Home* balloons and streamers, but he hardly notices. We'd tied them to the back of his TV chair, where they float above him in the little breeze from the air circulator. But he heads right for that chair and sinks into his old friend, without noticing. "Oh," he sighs. "Oh." He looks around. Everything as it was. The picture of the grandchildren he took one summer long ago, the television, the mirror over the couch, the light streaming in the sliding glass door, a fine day all around. He's been away a long time. Almost a month. He looks at the empty third chair, the door to my uncle's room closed for good.

"Hey, Dad, you made it," I say. You got out of there." Back at University House how glad they are to see him. How few ever make it back. My parents alone at last.

The first morning on their own, the residency nurse pays them a visit and insists that my father walk from his chair to the bathroom on his own. She wants to see if he's well enough to be home. Of course he's using his walker and he's weak from the illness, the hospital, the nursing home, his grief, and so he catches his foot on one of the legs of the walker, tumbles over, and crumples to the floor.

The nurse leaves my mother with a warning. The next morning my father falls again, just slides out of bed onto the floor. He's not hurt, but my mother cannot get him up, and of course my uncle's no longer there to help her, so by house rules, she must call 911. The nurse pays them another visit and lays it all out. It's only what my mother must have known in her deepest heart. If my father has another fall, he will not be able to stay there. He'll either have to go to a nursing home, or my mother will have to arrange for twenty-four-hour care until it's determined whether they can make it on their own. And so the gauntlet is thrown down. From now on, in order to stay with her, my father will have to pass tests that depend on strength he does not have. He has ninety days. He can only have twenty-four-hour care for ninety days; they aren't licensed to operate as a nursing home.

It doesn't take long for me to see what's at the end of those ninety days. And if my father can't stay at University House, where would he go? I want to scoop them up and take them both away from all sorrowing things. I want to take them both to our home and lock the door behind us, so nobody will ever say that time's run out and they have to leave. The children only come home on holidays now, so it's just Ed and me and plenty of room at home. I ask the nurse to put me in contact with a social worker, to help me figure things out.

So the social worker wants to see the house, of course, look us over. Our house. My husband built it twenty years ago during one of his summers off from teaching and coaching. I have always loved that he built it. It has always made me feel wrapped in love. We had bought a lot bordered on one side by a stretch of woods where the kids had all kinds of adventures—tree houses, forts, swings, and coyotes, raccoons, an occasional deer, and bats and owls that rustled and whirred in the dark. We'd hired Paul Marwang, an architect my husband had coached in football years ago. Paul was so creatively frustrated working for an industrial firm that he went a little crazy with our house. Ours was his first house; now he's so famous we couldn't afford to have him draw plans for a toolshed.

We were in love with light and asked him for windows everywhere. We designed the house around a loft with a skylight for my studies. I was working on my PhD then, and needed a place to work where I could also see what the kids were up to. Thus the cathedral ceilings and the cathedral dining room window. The upstairs has no walls to break things up, so you can look from the living room through the dining room and kitchen all the way to the sky wall at the other end of the house. When the trees are no more than leafless sculptures with no promise in sight, the thin light of winter comes through those windows with such a memory of spring, you believe in it still.

Plenty of room for everything, or so it seemed at the time—except for one incredibly tiny upstairs bathroom with no room for a person who needs a walker and an aide. And fourteen stairs leading downstairs to the bedrooms and another small bathroom. Seven stairs down, then a little landing to turn around in, and down seven more stairs. I wondered about those lifts or chairs that got people up and down, since by now my father could not manage any stairs at all. We would need two of them. But the wall by the second set of stairs was only a half wall, and would not support such weight. Plenty of rooms downstairs but no way to get there. Or back up. Looking at it through these new circumstances, my wondrous house seemed fraught with tragic shortcomings.

Outside, my husband had built a series of cascading decks leading from the back door off the kitchen, down to the deck just outside our bedroom, which holds the hot tub. Just a quick two-step from inside to outside, even in the coldest weather, into that hot frothy water to watch the moon rise up over those dark, wintry trees. Such a house. Such good fortune that we could live here, that my husband could have made such a thing.

The social worker looks things over, goes downstairs. "It's a wonderful house," she says. "You must love living here."

"I do," I say. "I've never taken it for granted. The water district bought all the property out back so we'll always have those woods."

We sit down on the couch by the sky wall, look out at the tree in the pale December light. I bring her tea.

"Is it possible?" I ask. I look out at the deck off the family room at the front of the house. A long time ago we'd thought about making that into another room. I wish we had.

As it turns out, she says what I already know in my heart: short of remodeling the house, there is no way my father could *reasonably* live here. I swim in that word. We could make do with a little swatch of the unreasonable for his sake.

I start to lay all this out for my mother, ticking down the list of things we could do to accommodate him.

"No," my mother says, stopping me in the middle of my tortured description. "We would never do this." She's thinking of our lives and how their needs would completely take them over. She's thinking of what it was like to have my grandmother live with them all those years.

My heart closes off just then, and I take her at her word. I don't try to persuade her that we could somehow make things work. My relief that it is not possible, that there is no ambiguity in this, makes me feel only a little guilty. My unsheltered guilt will come later. And so the search for a place for my father for the end of days begins.

The third fall happens when I'm at school. I don't know anything about how he'd slipped off the toilet, bruised his arm, how the medics had patched him up but determined he was all right, how the nurse had rushed up.

I jump when the phone rings. It's the middle of the afternoon and I'm in my office gathering materials for my last class of the day. I've stopped taking my cell phone everywhere I go. My father is safe at University House now. He's out of the danger zone of food stored at unsafe temperatures, slipups in medications, worse things I could not remember from the nursing home web site check list. When the phone rings I take a deep breath before I answer it.

It's my mother. "I just wanted to let you know Gary's living with us now," she says calmly.

Gary? Who's Gary?

It is a pronouncement. Something has been settled. I can hear the relief in her voice. She might as well have said we've adopted a son, because that's what he became in the brief two weeks he stayed with them.

Now my uncle's door that had been shut will be opened again. Someone else will sit in my uncle's TV chair, sleep in his bed, sit at his desk. The irony of that good fortune goes unspoken. Agency rules demand that health aides have a room of their own. So my parents have had three days. They have lived alone for three days out of the last forty years.

Gary answers the door wearing yellow rubber gloves, a dish towel hung over his right shoulder. He's wearing baggy green khakis and a damp white T-shirt. He's a bear of a man. He puts out his hand.

"Hi. I'm Gary."

It's shocking to see a stranger in my parents' apartment. This burly man, with the heavy forehead and heavy brows that shade his acute brown eyes, has come to save them. He looks a little Neanderthal in that way some people do. But that look does not hide his intelligence or sensibility. Gary can discuss the economy. He has a son he sees now and then, a business venture that has failed in some unnamed way. He says he subs for short stretches for the home health care agency every so often to give him humility. It reminds him of the cycle of life, of the plenitude of life even at the end. We all fall in love with Gary. For a time we believe he actually is an angel.

Gary believes in bleach. Gary believes in bleach like others believe in prayers and vitamins and crystals and incantations. Gary tears through the apartment, yellow rubber gloves up to his elbows. My parents have housekeeping services every week, so I can't imagine what more needs to be cleaned. We never see him when he isn't in the middle of cleaning something. My mother's often perplexed, as we all are, as to how all that cleaning could make such a mess. Piles of things everywhere. On the kitchen table, the counters, even the couch. My mother has kept that apartment neat as the proverbial pin. It's as though things have unsorted themselves from the nooks and crannies and shelves and drawers of my mother's careful management into growing piles of laundry, magazines, newspapers, towels, cleaning supplies.

Gary brings his own food and cooks vats of broccoli and cauliflower. He eats plates of it. He says it's his new way to lose weight. The smell permeates the apartment and mixes with the bleach. It's all right. Everything's all right now.

Overnight the cough my father had carried home with him from Bessie Burton has turned into bronchitis and some mysterious stomach ailment. Food stored at unsafe temperatures comes to mind. Then my father starts throwing up, and sits propped up in his TV chair with a bowl and towel and the dry heaves. And then violent diarrhea while he struggles to get up out of his chair and onto his walker. Then my mother gets the dry heaves, either in sympathy, or from something she's caught from my father, or from Bessie Burton. She sits in the TV chair in the living room with a bowl and towel in her lap too, while Gary rushes from one to the other. Maybe that explains all that bleach and the yellow rubber gloves. No one but Gary could have ever handled this. "It was quite a time," Gary says, "your father going at both ends." He says it with a little laugh, as though to say, it's all right. It's just what the body does. There is no shame here.

Gary talks to my father, not around him, or through my mother. He asks my father's permission. "Homer, is it all right if I give you your shower now?" This bear of a man has a gentle touch and a gift for knowing exactly what to do. He straightens my father in his chair, adjusts a pillow here and there, bathes him from head to toe. He knows things. He knows about food at unsafe temperatures. He knows when the pharmacy sends my father the wrong medication. He knows what to do when my father chokes. He knows that the tips of my father's toes turning red is not a good sign. "You need a support here for the blankets at the end of the bed," he tells my mother. "I don't like how this looks." My father had been hospitalized the year before for an infected toe. One of the nurses had casually mentioned amputation. But Gary will save him. He will know what to look out for. My parents have forgotten about the short stretch. My parents think he'll stay with them forever. Having Gary means they can stay together.

Ed and I invite him to our Thanksgiving. Gary says he'd like to come to Thanksgiving because his job is to take care of Homer and he wants to be sure everything goes all right. And since his son will be with his mother, he has nowhere special to go anyway.

My father's entourage arrives. Gary and my husband help my father into the house, and he clumps his way on his walker toward the easy chair in the corner, while Gary reaches around to guide him into the chair. Alex, the dog, has never seen Gary before. She doesn't know he's an angel. My dog, who has always loved my father best, lunges at Gary and grabs the arm that is helping my father. He isn't hurt, but it surprises him. It surprises us all. *Alex, no!* Her ears flatten for a moment, as she takes on that chastised look, and backs off a couple of feet. But then her ears go right back up and she stands her ground, watching. She growls a low, soft growl. Well. This will never do. There is enough to worry about without wondering if our eighty-five-pound dog will go for the throat next time. *Shame on you, Alex.* You ought to know better than that. Obviously, she's no judge of character. Or maybe she is. Maybe she was growling at his otherworldliness. Maybe this was proof of who he really was. Animals are so earthbound, so connected to the things of the body, to weather and sky. She's never done anything like this before. Of course, she herself is preternatural. She can read our minds. We've seen it often enough to respect her intelligence and something else we could never quite name. But now she is banished to the backyard in the rain, though not without the greatest of protests. She will not be left out when she has work to do. She wails all through the evening, hunched against the backdoor.

Then my son, Chris, arrives. He's barely a week out of knee surgery for a torn ACL. He'd torn it before, but he's been gracious about his bad luck, though now, as he hobbles through the front door on crutches, Maureen and Robb bringing up the rear, he's practically in tears from the pain. It's his first trip out, first trip down the perilous stairs of the apartment, then stretched out in the backseat of the car, the pain meds not having kicked in yet.

"I'm gonna throw up," he says. "I never should have come." It is the voice of despair. He edges carefully onto the couch, props up his leg, puts his head back, shuts his eyes, and lets the meds do their work at last. I try to tell myself what a great story this will all make someday, how funny it will be—the kid with the leg, the dog, Gary the angel.

Courtney has been here all afternoon, helping us set up. She goes outside to comfort the dog. My daughter understands why Alex is banned from the house but can hardly bear her wails. We can all hear the wind driving the rain against the house, and think about her howling and scratching at the door. It's the sound of Alex's despair at being outside the lighted circle where she belongs, because she can't save us now. She wails again. It's the sound at the edge of our hearts anyway. And besides, she'll keep this up until we let her back in. I think about my uncle and the wail with no sound, and The Wailer at Bessie Burton, and find this isn't such a comic story after all.

But eventually we gather around the dining room table. Chris is himself again. The meds have done their job, and he's calm now, even starts to joke. He's all set up next to the dining room table in the recliner with a tray of food on his lap. My father is seated at the head of the table, as always. Our usual mode is to ask him to say grace, but now we fear he will break down. "Let's just not say a blessing this year," I say to my husband. My mother is consulted. It's a conspiracy among us. So it is agreed that my husband will briefly gives thanks for love and for food and for all those we have always loved, an oblique reference to the dead so recently with us. I can't tell if my father notices this side step, but it is the first and only time it will ever occur.

My mother sits next to my father, so she can serve him food, cut his meat. I'm sitting next to my mother, playing jack-in-the-box, Betty Crocker on speed. Gary is sitting across from my mother on the other side of my father. He's like an old family member we haven't seen for years. He takes up the place that would have been my uncle's. My husband is at the foot of the table, and the kids tucked in between—our daughter, our sons, and our daughter-in-law.

We have made it a feast for the eye as well as the heart. The rapture of this season coming to an end spread out before us. We are in love with color. The autumn centerpiece, with the orange, yellow, gold-tinged leaves, tiny red berries, red apples, pears, plums. And in white porcelain dishes—yams, beets, cranberries, creamed spinach, mashed potatoes, turkey, gravy, apple pie, pumpkin pie, vanilla ice cream, raspberries, slices of cheddar cheese. We will eat and eat to know we are alive, while death for the moment has vanished behind some fickle cloud. For a brief season the empty chair is filled. We take pictures, sure that Gary, angel that he is, will be invisible to the camera eye. And that is how we made our way through Thanksgiving, our faces in the rain-spattered cathedral window, tilting and bobbing in the light.

After dinner we sit around the living room, the slanting rain, the wail of the dog counterpoint to the pleasant faces we have assumed for the day. We listen to Gary tell stories, grateful for someone with something to say—his strange, eclectic life, a little about his family, broken in some irrevocable way, his experience as a small business owner, though what business it was or how it failed, we never knew. I remember how easy we were with each other, and how much we wanted him to love us. It didn't have to be much. Just enough so he would never leave my parents and their lives could go on. And why not? He'd already dropped out of the sky. All right, he didn't have to actually be an angel. And if not love, then kindness. That's what we most wanted from everyone who ever touched my father now.

All the competing urgencies I felt toward my father's great need of me vanished like mist, and left only an infinite tenderness. He was becoming sacred before my very eyes. Yet to go about the practical business of keeping him on this earth, that luminous sense of him could only be borne for so long. You could only bear to see that radiant quality in flashes. A full view of it would strike you dead. Your astonished hands would hang at your sides. Your mouth would shape into wordlessness. You'd be no good at all. And besides, the earthly pull of him was still too great, and you were days, months, *years* from ever giving him up.

Then one day Gary was gone, never to return. His two weeks were up. The day Gary left and Zinda arrived was a day of mourning. It was like a death in the family all over again. By now Gary had become like a son. He filled up the room. His ample presence said I'll take care of you no matter what. Now he was gone and my parents never recovered from losing him. My father would have been carted back to Bessie Burton, or some such place, if Gary hadn't shown up, and they knew it.

Zinda was from Uganda. He was small and shy and uncertain, and spoke so quietly and with such an accent my parents could not understand him. They didn't believe he could take care of them. But it wouldn't have mattered who the agency sent after Gary. It was December when Zinda came, but Zinda wore shorts and went around in his bare feet. Of course, my parents kept the thermostat turned up to eighty. Zinda was kind and honest, and as I pointed out to my father, read the Bible and listened to the same religious TV programs he did, which ought to have made up for something, but it didn't. Zinda was initially too shy to tell my mother what he wanted for meals. As it turned out, all he really wanted were hot dogs. He ate them for breakfast, lunch, and dinner. Zinda stayed in my uncle's room, waiting to be needed. That's what my parents were paying him for. To help with getting up and getting down. He did no cooking or cleaning or bleaching.

Zinda was a small, quiet presence who lived in the shadow of my parents' lives, who gave them far more privacy than Gary ever did. He moved silently on bare feet to my father's side on a whisper or a sigh, learning finally to anticipate what was not yet spoken, an ebony angel who floated about the apartment along the edges of my parents' lives in a tender, almost poignant way.

But for all his kindness, Zinda was so inexperienced that my mother let him go. So one day Zinda left and Malek arrived. Malek had two ex-wives back in the Philippines, an indeterminate number of children, and complicated domestic and legal problems. Smoking was banned throughout the building, but Malek would grab a smoke now and then in my uncle's bedroom, though to his credit he usually sat at the desk by an open window. Malek asked my mother for money just to tide him over until the next paycheck, something that would have gotten him fired if my mother had ever reported it. She gave it to him, then asked me if I thought she should hide her money. So we hid her cash inside a big dictionary on the floor of their bedroom closet.

But at least they could understand Malek. And he was big enough to handle my father in the more complicated ways he needed now. For Malek, I bought Hungry Man dinners—Fried Chicken, Pot Roast, Chicken Fried Steak.

Through those weeks Malek was there, my father's problems doubled—first one thing then another, and after each fall, illness, trip to the ER, he left a little more of himself behind. He began to have episodes of confusion, and more times of garbled speech. A sentence would start out just fine and then derail a few words into it, ending in kind of train wreck at the end. He seemed philosophical about it, but it must have frightened him. He'd start to talk and we'd nod and nod—of course we know what you mean, Dad, we get it, no problem. And most of the time we more or less did. Though it must have been alarming to feel the words running out the sides of his mouth, down his shirt, and watch us reaching out to catch them. *Impedimenta*, he called himself increasingly those last days. It was his way of saying *burden, millstone, albatross.*

We were well into February by now and those ninety days were running out. His nights became disrupted by all kinds of things—sleeplessness, constipation, aches and pains and mysterious symptoms that came and went—then toward morning he would fall so deeply into sleep he could not be wakened. My father was becoming too much even for Malek. "I wish he would just let go in his sleep," my mother confided to me a few days before my father would quit the apartment for good. "Before he ever has to leave." So because I could not stop it, my parents' life together came to an end.

The Long Goodbye

It's Valentine's Day at University House. My husband and I are sitting with my parents at the big oak table in the center of the dining room for the Valentine's Day dinner, waiting for the buffet line to thin out. Then I take my father's plate and go through the line. Prime rib, roasted potatoes, asparagus, a little salad, tiramisu for dessert. Tomorrow my father will say goodbye to all this, the beautiful lobby, the Dale Chihuly sculptures in the library, the baby grand, the gourmet food—goodbye to my mother, goodbye to everything, to go to the nursing home forever. My mother will stay in their apartment and my father will go where he will get the twenty-four-hour care he needs. My father always said that you'd broken the back of winter once you reached Valentine's Day. It was always his marker for getting through the worst of it. So today is Valentine's Day, and the worst of it is just beginning.

No one stops to say goodbye. They either don't know they'll never see my father again, or don't know what to say if they do. All except for Ginny, who has asked to sit with us for the last supper, though none of us is calling it that. "I won't say goodbye," she whispers to me at the end of the meal, as she turns down the hall. She's pushing a walker and trailing an oxygen tank.

For a minute I wonder what she's thinking as she makes her way back to her room. One more friend come and gone. I wonder briefly what it's like to live on the edge like that, but then turn my attention to my parents, who will say goodbye tonight to their life together.

"They're kicking me out," my father had said earlier in the week. And in fact they are. He cannot stay where he is, needing twenty-four-hour care. "Would they let me stay if I could walk on crutches?" he'd said. Or walk on water, he might as well have added. He can only use the walker for short distances and then only if someone is holding his belt. He can't get from his walker to his chair or the bed or the toilet by himself anymore. And he's becoming too much for the health aide. He's been too much for my mother for way too long now.

"Would they let me stay if I offered to be the chaplain?"

"Homer, they don't even have a chaplain," my mother says. "This isn't a religious place." But there is no translation.

"Can you come with me?" he finally asks her. No, she can't, and all the reasons why cannot be explained into understanding. All he knows is that he will be without her. He has been in love with her his whole life and now everything between them will change for good.

I wondered what it would it be like—to be banished like that. Boarding school, or military school, or jail, with no time off for good behavior, no outside privileges for the holidays. Or maybe an endless summer camp with activities you hadn't the slightest interest in. Or the nut house. That was probably closer to the truth of it.

That night after the Valentine's dinner, he took his last "hall walk": a slow, two-step shuffle with his walker down the hall, with Malek holding on to the back of his belt and pushing a wheelchair behind him if he wavered or slipped to the side.

"Homer, you don't want to go there. You don't want to do it," Malek had said. "I know about that place. It's a terrible place." I knew what Malek was doing. He only wanted to keep this cushy job. But this was what my father heard the night before his life with my mother would come to an end.

My father knew better than to think of it as rehab. He'd been to rehab and he knew the difference. This was not Bessie Burton for a short stay. This was Ida Culver for the long haul. Three days earlier I'd taken him to see his doctor at the medical center for the last time. He'd have a new doctor now, someone assigned to the nursing home by his insurance company—a doctor we never saw, who never, as far as we know, actually saw him.

"Will I ever get out of there?" he'd asked Dr. Featherston, his regular doctor. I'd called ahead and talked to the nurse, said how depressed he was, so be sure to give him some hope, a pep talk.

"I don't think so, Homer," Dr. Featherston said. "I don't think you will." Was this some kind of demented geriatric tough love? I wanted to shout. But I said nothing. Nothing. Nothing.

"Well, I guess it's the end of the trail," my father had said as we were getting lunch in the hospital cafeteria. "No, no, no," I'd said way too brightly. "This isn't the end of the trail, this is just the beginning. They're going to get you back into shape, Dad, get you moving again." The physical therapist at Ida Culver had worked out a plan in advance. Three times a week. Walks in the hall, stretching, leg lifts lying in bed. It made me hope Dr. Featherston was wrong. That there was a minor miracle or two around some bend in the road. But as things turned out, by the time the physical therapist was on board the second week, my father had had a setback and couldn't even stand up by himself, let alone go for a walk.

How my mother and father said goodbye that last night I do not know. All I know is that here they were being wrenched apart after all those years, and I couldn't do a thing to stop it. But then as these things go, he finally gets all checked in to the nursing home, his pajamas in the drawer, his room fixed up to look like home. I rush to the nursing home from work to be with him on his first night at Ida Culver. I take the elevator up to the second floor where the lifers stay, people who will not be going home. The elevator has a funny smell I can't at first identify. The lobby did not smell like this. The elevator up to the rehab floor did not smell like this either. But I learn soon enough what that smell is. Nothing mysterious, just the smells of the body saying goodbye and food gone bad and Lysol and floral deodorizer, the death-sweet coverup, the odor of chrysanthemums a short way down the road. Now it begins, I say to myself.

The elevator doors open onto the nurses' station, but there is no one behind the desk, no one in the hall. Everything is cast in an eerie, yellowy light. A rush of fear washes over me. When I'd looked this place over weeks ago, there were plenty of people around. I make my way to my father's assigned room. And there he is, in his wheelchair, hunched over a little inspirational magazine he's trying to read by the pale bed light. "How God Gave Me Power to Walk Again" is the article he's reading. For months now he has dreamed he can walk. I dream it too, only when he throws his walker aside and steps back into his life, he takes a shaky step or two into the street and slips and hits his head on the concrete just outside my reaching arms.

"Hi, Dad," I say.

"Hi, Pill," he says and his face lights up like he hasn't seen me for years, like I'm not the one who put him here. Soon, our conversation is interrupted by a screaming from next door. A man in the next room is shouting from his bed, waving his hands in the air. His gown has slipped off his thin white shoulder. "Help! Help!" he shouts when he sees me standing in the doorway. I walk into his room, over to his bed.

"What do you need?" I say. My heart is racing. Not a nurse or aide in sight. I'd only seen this place by day, and I start to imagine the horrors of what happens here after dark. I'm ready to scoop my father up and get him out of here.

"Help!" the old guy shouts again, looks at me standing at the foot of the bed.

"What do you need?" I say again.

"I want meat! Hamburger! Sausage! Pork! Bologna! Bacon!"

"I'm sorry," I say, "I can't help you." I back away and make my exit. Now I've met my father's next-door neighbor.

"The loony bin," my father says when I come back into the room. He's trying to make a joke, but he's frightened behind the smile. We're in for it now, I think to myself.

The other bed in the room is empty. "Have you met your roommate yet?" I ask. He doesn't quite know how to answer. Such great hopes for the roommate, whoever he is: a new friend, a chess partner, a buddy, a soulmate, and if not an identical twin, a brother. At the very least, someone who could help take my mother's place in decent conversation, discuss the economy or politics or history. As I turn to leave, I see my father's roommate trying to get his wheelchair back into the room but it catches in the doorway. "Can I help you?"

He grabs my arm and whispers hoarsely in a long-drawn-out voice: "Get me *out* of here!" Out of this chair? Out of this room? Out of this place? Out of this life? Marlon, the nearly silent roommate who never kept any personal belongings in that room, who lay on his right side on the top of his bed in his clothes waiting to die. Marlon sank our spirits. But it was all right. By then my friendly, garrulous father had run out of things to say.

We decorated my father's side of the room to show that this man was loved. This man's family was paying attention and would permit no mistakes. My daughter has feng shui-ed the room and determined that the window is the water side of the room, and hung a blue and green fish mobile with satin ribbons like seaweed flickering in the breeze from the heating vent across the room. We have put great hopes in this room with a view. We haven't tucked him into a dark, forgotten corner after all. How it comforts us to walk into the room and see that light.

My daughter has put up her PETA calendar of animals rescued from experimental horrors, which has found some echo in her heart. Behind the bed we've hung a couple of my father's historical photographs—Lincoln's log cabin, the statue of Benedict Arnold's leg. Conversation starters for the nurses and aides. "So you took these pictures, huh?" And he'd be pulled back into his life, reminded of who he was. "Some of my historical pictures are in the *Encyclopaedia Britannica*," he could say, though I don't know if he ever did. He could barely remember this other self. The photographs were his only proof. My principal memory of these photographic trips was of my mother trying to keep me occupied while my father waited for the light to turn just so. Light was light. It all looked the same to me.

I'd thought of putting up the picture of him shaking hands with Ronald Reagan, but he hated Reagan. Yet my father was a party man, so he eventually and reluctantly supported him, although in the picture you can see my father is forcing the smile. When he was in rehab trying to learn how to write again, he practiced on his favorite slogan—NOW IS THE TIME FOR EVERY GOOD MAN TO COME TO THE AID OF HIS PARTY. Better to be shaking hands with Gerald Ford, because in this picture my father's proud as he can be; he's striding into the picture ready to embrace his little moment of fame. In that picture you can see what an athletic man Ford was, despite all his well-documented tumbles and slips. Or maybe the picture with Nelson Rockefeller, whom my father admired greatly. Back at University House, those pictures are framed and biding their time on the wall above my father's chair—Rockefeller to the left, Ford in the center, and Reagan far to the right, my mother's little joke. But in this tiny half room at Ida Culver, there is no space for this triptych, and nobody to take the time to stand back and appreciate the irony. On the other hand, someone might ask him how these pictures came to be and my father could talk about his life in politics, and how once he'd spent the day with John Kennedy, when he was running for president.

My father was an artist in black-and-white: a series of photographs of seagulls in flight; sunflowers in a chiaroscuro of dark and light; the Old North Church, and Old Ironsides, with lines so clean and precise they could be an artist's rendering; the Liberty Bell in such ravishing bronze it looks strong enough for the ages, belied only by that crack up the middle; and antebellum mansions caught in light casting lacy shadows through a flush of trees. From Boston to Florida, history played out before him, each place loved twice-over, by one in love with history, one in love with light. My favorite photograph: a Civil War cannon perched on a high, stony outcropping overlooking a vast landscape wrapped in such liminal haze it could be any terrain, any war. The cannon is locked up by the chain keeping it silent for good. It's winter or very early spring because in the upper right-hand corner you can see wintry branches with the very beginning of buds. I don't know why it's my favorite, except for what it tells of my father: who would have thought to wait for such unsheltered light, so soft, so otherworldly.

Just to prove to him that everything is as it was, we gather to take him out to dinner that first weekend, to a Mexican restaurant nearby. "See Dad? We can still all get together and do things." But my father is stunned to be out in the world. It reminds him of all he's lost. "I wish Henry were here," he tells my mother.

"Henry *hated* Mexican food," she says sharply. Of course she knows what he means. My father is remembering their Saturday lunches, the three of them making their way up the block to Beso del Sol, the Tombstone burrito, the little bowls of salsa. My mother is angry that he's still so pulled by him and not by her.

The second weekend we do the same, only now my father is accompanied by a catheter and a bladder bag. Something had happened during that week. He'd become disoriented, frightened, didn't know night from day. Too weak to get up to use the bathroom. Dehydration maybe, or a little stroke. I thought it was his broken heart, and there's no fix for that. But they'd rehydrated him, adjusted his meds, and he seemed to recover, except that now it took two aides to get him in and out of bed. Now they couldn't get him up and to the bathroom in time. By the time they'd finally answered his call button it was often too late. So they'd asked for permission to insert a catheter and my mother and I had given it. But my father was afraid of catheters and for good reason. He remembered what had happened before.

"I hate catheters," Carrie the nurse had said. Apparently there were dangers to catheters she did not explain. She seemed to think you turned a corner with a catheter and you could never get back. I didn't see her logic and thought it would just make things easier all around, since it was so torturous now getting my father out of bed in time, and it bypassed the ignominy of diapers. "I know what happened before, Homer." She'd read my father's hospital notes. "I know how to do this," she said. And she did. And so from then on, the bladder bag hung unceremoniously by the side of the bed.

"Couldn't you paint on a daffodil, or at least a smiley face?" my mother had said to the kids. She knew it was there for the duration, and why not? And though it would've made a great joke, none of us ever did. We all tried not to look at it, or to think of it as a permanent attachment. Our eyes played trickster with that bladder bag those last weeks, that betrayal of the body we did not want to see, let alone touch. When to our mutual embarrassment the inside things came shamefully outside, and there was cleaning up to do, we were inclined to look away.

By the third week, the PT guy has warned us not to try to take my father out anymore. It's taking two aides to move him now as it is. So the next Sunday we gather in the little family room at the end of the hall with the Mexican food we brought in. But by then my father has lost his appetite for Mexican food. He's pretty much lost his appetite altogether.

A few weeks later, my daughter and I bring the dog in to cheer him up. We don't ask permission or anything. She's so big we can't exactly sneak her in, so we're just going to take our chances. We keep her on a tight leash and quickly make our way out of the elevator and down the hall to my father's room. Marlon is asleep on his side and takes no notice. My father's asleep too. Alex goes right to him and licks his arm. He startles into waking and smiles. "Alex! I didn't know you could come here." My father looks at me.

"Oh, we just brought her. We didn't ask anybody."

My father worries about breaking the rules.

"It's okay, Dad, she won't hurt anything."

Then Alex discovers the bladder bag and such richness of smells she forgets my father altogether, perks up her ears, wags her tail at everything.

I wonder what she knows from these earthly smells, or if she smells death around this corner or that. It's a short visit, but we have come. We have come to say goodbye.

"I don't like it here," my father says to me one day. "How long do I have to stay here?"

For a minute I can't say anything at all. Then I say, "That depends, Dad." He's a child now, in many ways, and has no way of knowing what's best for him. I don't either, anymore. So I say in all truth, "As soon as you can get on your feet." By God, yes, as soon as you can do that I'm wheeling you out of here as fast as I can. We'll make some spectacular getaway.

I'm sitting by my dad in a half moon of wheelchairs in the activity room. It's exercise class. Everybody raises one arm, then the other; one leg, then the other; claps, stomps their feet, tosses a giant blue beach ball. My dad, who'd been a college athletic director, a basketball coach, raises one shaky arm on the first exercise then sits there with his hands in his lap. "See, Dad? It's your workout." Then the recreation director puts the beach ball down and claps her hands. It's singing time she says. "You love to sing," I remind him. "You have a wonderful voice." But there is no piano accompaniment, no tape on the tape deck, no razzmatazz, no jive. Just her chirping voice carrying along a few tremulous female voices and one completely flat male voice, which turns out to be Marlon's, the only other man in the room. I set an example, join in.

You are my sunshine, my only sunshine.

I steal glances at my father, who cannot remember how to sing. He's just sitting there staring into his lap.

You make me happy when skies are gray
You'll never know dear how much I love you.
Please don't take my sunshine away.

Then he looks at me as tears slide down his face. My mother. That's what we've done, all right. We've taken her away.

Some who work here are angels on this earth. Jim, the nurse who plays piano jazz during dinner and watches over my dad's medications; Lisa, who tells me to go ahead and cry, it's grief work you're doing.

Others are not: there is Jay, the red-haired nurse's aide, with the Day-Glo burst of energy, which my mother loves and I hate. "Homer, how *are* you today? We're gonna get you back on your *feet*." And Carrie, the charge nurse, who bustles into the room and waves a form in my mother's face. "You didn't sign this," she barks.

"I think I signed everything," my mother says. She's subdued now, and just stands there by my father, who's sitting in his wheelchair pointed toward the window, his back to us. My mother can't figure out what Carrie's saying.

"You know," Carrie said, "the form that tells me what to do if I come in here some morning and find him not breathing. Do we do CPR on him and then haul him to the hospital? Or do you want this to be it?" I have no idea if my father has heard this, but when I look back at him he's slumped to the side of his wheelchair.

"No CPR," my mother finally whispers.

Carrie, with the pear-shaped body, her heavy thighs in white polyester that sound her comings and goings. Her strawberry blonde hair hangs down her back in long ropy curls. I want to smack her. She could have said, "Grace, can you step into the hall for a minute? We need to talk." I wondered if this was carelessness of the most egregious form, or some perverse kind of nursing home tough-love therapy. I wondered what her life was like to bring her to such carelessness. I had no idea what it took from her to see people at the end of the road day after day, the outcome on this floor never a surprise. But I also never forgot her skill with the catheter.

That winter after my uncle had died and my father had gone to the nursing home, I was finishing a long novel I was writing set in Cuba. I had been working on it for a very long time and was coming to the end of it. The beat and thrum of Havana, that blue heartbreak of a sky, the arc of the Malecón that curved around the city, that astonishing light—all were as far away as I could get from Ida Culver. I wrote the ending to that novel during those same winter weeks, and have never stopped believing that the eroticism of those last chapters came from living so close to death. Through the dark, sleety rain of February and March and the false promises of April I wrote like a woman drowning. I brought my laptop to my father's room and set it up on my dad's bed tray, put on my headset, and typed a few fragmented paragraphs now and then while my father slept. It kept me in the room when otherwise I'd have gone running down the hall and out the door. That winter my writing was the only safe place there was.

"What's wrong with that rabbit?" my father says, just now noticing the irregularities of the poster animals in the PETA calendar on his bulletin board across the room. My daughter had just turned the calendar from March to April, and there is the April animal of the month—a white rabbit with an irregular black patch of fur around its left eye.

"It's an animal rescued from a lab," I explain.

"What lab?" he says. He doesn't know what I'm talking about, and so we move on. It's all right. Some things you don't have to know anymore. We'd gotten through the last days of the month of the cat, through the long rainy month of the dog, and we were beginning the month of the rabbit. It was a new way of marking time. What were months and weeks anyway? There were only days and hours.

These days it doesn't matter anymore if his socks don't match or if the shirt he's wearing isn't his, or his dinner is a little cold or they forget to wash behind his ears. None of this matters now, yet once it seemed to matter tragically, even though none of it seemed to matter to him. Earlier all these things would have been grievous, unsupportable errors, signs of far greater, more dangerous failings.

Days go by that chart a steady, inexorable decline. Then it's Easter, and my mother has gotten special permission to go over to the other side—to take my father from the nursing home to the beautiful dining room in the adjacent retirement center overlooking the water, where she's reserved a table for all of us. She's told the staff to be sure he's all dressed up in his camel blazer and nice blue shirt and dress shoes. But when we get there at 11, he's been sitting in his wheelchair all ready to go for over two hours and his back is throbbing. My husband and son manage to get him out of the wheelchair and back into bed, something we'll just have to reverse in a little while.

Everybody brings flowers. We goof around, take crazy pictures, anything for a laugh. We sit around a long table. The only one missing is my uncle. My father eats shrimp dipped in hot cocktail sauce. That's all he wants. It's the one thing he can still taste. He doesn't say a word. He looks around. All these people, going about their lives. It's all unreal to him, this new setting, people all dressed up, moving around on their own. They'd never know he'd come from the other side but for the wheelchair. We fill our plates again and again. We have never been so hungry. The mountains are off in the distance; the water shimmers in the sun. Angels hover. Send in the clowns.

We know what this is. This afternoon my father will go into hospice. What this means we're not exactly sure, except for the new hydraulic mattress and the new ergonomic wheelchair he'll be getting. All things for the long haul, when of course by now we all know there will be no long haul. Then it's our appointed time and we're ushered into a little windowless side room, furnished for such last things, and listen while the hospice representative explains all the intricacies of what hospice will and will not do. My father tries to follow it all, but cannot.

"Homer, do you have any questions?" the hospice rep finally asks. Her name is Ann too.

My father's eyes are brimming. He looks at us and then at her. "Does this mean I'm ready to croak?"

She's a little startled at his word choice, but goes right on ahead. "No, Homer. It just means you'll be more comfortable. Everything that's done now will be for that."

He looks at my mother. "Grace? What do you think?"

My mother can hardly speak. "It's a good idea, Homer," she says. She does not look at him.

"Okay," he shrugs. He's tired beyond speaking now and wants to go back to his room.

"You can eat whatever you want now, Dad," I say, as I wheel him back home.

"I can?" After decades of diabetic prohibitions it's a startling concept. Trouble is, he's lost his appetite long ago. But there will be no more tests, no more needle jabs, no more trips by cabulance to his doctors downtown, no more blood transfusions, no more experimental treatments. I recite the perilous advantages. And no more IV hydration, no more antibiotics, no more rescues. After so many rescues, it's a concept I can't believe in. But soon he's fast asleep in his bed by the window he never looks out, and we gather up our things. We put the sad little Easter lily on the nightstand and say a goodbye he does not hear. We have done the deed. And the last Easter has come to an end.

On the drive home I think of my father's life, so distant from him now. I think of all the students over the years who had loved him and all the needy ones who attached themselves to him, like the boy who in his senior year in college found out that his father was not his father, that he had been adopted as an infant, whom my father talked out of quitting school. Or the girl with such terrible acne she couldn't look you in the eye, and how my father got her to a dermatologist and paid the bills.

On Monday afternoon, a week before the true end of things, they suddenly transfer my father to another room in another wing, and another set of nurses and aides. My father's labs have just come back. He's been diagnosed with a staph infection for which there is no cure, and they want him to room with the only other patient on the floor with the same thing. My father will share a room with Lloyd, who has that staph infection too, and Clarence would be moved into my father's room with Marlon. I remembered Carrie saying how much she hated catheters. But we *want* him to have a catheter, we all said. Anything for his comfort, since by now it was practically taking a forklift to get him up onto his feet. Now I knew why. Just another entry site for infection, dummy.

Monday night I find him in his new room in a bed by the door, slumped under the dim yellow light that casts a thin shadow across his sleeping face. It's getting dark now, and I can see lights in the distance out the window on the other side of the room. A curtain is pulled around Lloyd's bed, a futon or something like it, on the floor. Ravel's "Concerto for the Left Hand" is playing on my father's little radio tucked against his pillow. Ah, yes, I think. The left hand. It was a good pinch hitter these last couple of years since the stroke.

He wakes up when I touch his face. "What can I do for you, Dad? A little soft ice cream? Some cold water? Now you can have anything you want." Now, after years of denial, he can have every sweet thing he ever wanted.

"I'm so thirsty," he says. "I don't think they know I'm here." And maybe they don't. There is too much going on in the bed across the room. Lloyd is making a huge commotion, groaning and yelling and retching. Curiously, my father does not seem to be bothered by all this. I press the HELP button, then finally go out into the hall. Can somebody please help this poor man?

Jay, the red-haired nurse, finally comes in. "Oh yeah, he's been doing that all day. We just get him cleaned up and there he goes again." Then I realize it's blood he's throwing up. "We've been trying to get hold of his doctors all day."

I look at my father. We can't keep this up forever.

"He's a full code, if you can believe it," Jay says. "I wouldn't want to do CPR on *that* chest. I'd break every rib he's got." I should have gone over to say something, some word of comfort, some human touch, because there Lloyd was in that darkened circle of the room on the floor.

"I'm so thirsty," my dad says again. "Could you get me something to drink?" But this I cannot do. I hold the plastic cup to his mouth and he takes a sip and chokes and chokes and I think he's never going to breathe again. He is unremembering how to swallow. I run out into the hall, try to grab someone again. The hall has gone dark, except for the yellowy glow from the exit light. "Can somebody please come and help?" I say. I go back into my father's room. "I'm just so thirsty. Couldn't I have a little water?" I burst into tears, then calm down and touch his face.

"Can I do anything else?" I am remembering my uncle. "I'm afraid about the water." He opens his eyes and takes me in.

"Just love me," he whispers. I pick up a washrag and wash his face with cool water. I can't stop the tears from slipping down my face.

"Dad, I'll be right back," I say. I get out into the hall as fast as I can and make it to the end of the hall to the couch by the window. I lean over and put my head in my hands and sob. I can feel my heart coming apart inside my chest. It's hard to breathe. We are in hell. I know this light at the end of the hall has not turned red, but in my memory it seems like it. Suddenly there is a hand on my shoulder and someone is sitting down beside me. It's Lisa, the charge nurse on this new wing.

"It's good to cry," she says. "It's good for you."

"Oh," I say, "I don't want to cry in front of him."

"It tells him you love him."

"He's eighty-seven years old." I shake my head. I think how lucky I've been to have had him so long already, how ungrateful I am to be so sad.

"I know he's old," I say, "but he doesn't feel old to me."

"That much more of him to lose, not less. Our culture has no name for such loss." She takes my hand. "You're trembling," she says.

"I'm so scared," I say. "I don't know if I can do this."

"But here you are anyway."

"Not at night. I can't stay at night."

"There's the moon," she says. I turn around to see a golden moon hanging just above the trees.

"I wish I could believe in it," I say. "Such beauty."

"You can," she says. "Even here."

I turn back around to the yellow-lit hallway. "He's so thirsty and I can't seem to do it right. He keeps choking."

"I know something you can do." So she takes me to the fridge in the little kitchen off the nurse's station. She shows me the shelf with rows of clear plastic cups filled with something that looks suspiciously like gravy. It's called Thick-It.

"This will be easier for him than water. You can get him some anytime you want. Pretty soon he won't be thirsty. It's not painful to go without water. It often produces euphoria." It's a thought I hold on to all week.

We sit on the couch for a little longer without speaking, while she holds my hand. Suddenly we aren't in hell anymore.

Then in the middle of the night, long after I'd gone home, they take Lloyd away forever.

The next morning I'm there early. I have canceled my classes for the duration. I make the turn into his room and there it is before me. A private room at last. A flash of Puget Sound in the sun through the trees, the Olympics, snow-capped and imperious in the far distance, the sun shining on everything. And not one window, but a whole wall of windows. We have it all to ourselves. They will not move someone in with him now.

I sit down and pat his arm. He opens his eyes wide to take me in with a look that can only be called luminous. "We don't need words now, do we," he whispers.

"No, we don't," I say.

There is no break in time now. It spreads around him like a shimmery dream. Oh, to see your face again, outside the falling dreams. Our visits those last days must have been like mirages, our faces wavering in the light above the bed, one minute there, the next gone, then in an eyeblink back again. We come and go, trying to keep the threads of our lives from unraveling, living in communal suspended breath. He's becoming translucent now, transfigured. His face is filled with radiance, his eyes are full of light. I am memorizing his face. No. He is memorizing mine. So this is what the agony was for—this tenderness of the long goodbye where everything but love is falling away.

Those last days my father did not want to be touched, though he'd always loved it before. He'd draw his arm away or turn his head a little from my hand. I remember what Susan, my uncle's ICU nurse, had said when I asked after my uncle, who did the same thing. "He's entering the *death fugue*. What you see when you look at him is not what he's experiencing. He's not really in his body like you think. He's someplace else now and doesn't want to be called back."

"Do you want me to touch you?" I ask my father, just to make sure.

He shakes his head. No. No.

On Wednesday evening my cousin Carol flies in from California. She's an orphan now and wants to say goodbye to my father, whom she has always loved. I'm glad there's someone here I'm connected to by blood. Our mothers were sisters. We had the same grandparents. I say these things over to myself. I'm so glad to see her when she steps off the plane. We're going to drive directly to the nursing home so we both can tuck my father in for the night. On the way I tell her about the switched rooms, how he's doing. "You know he looks really good," I say. "He's lost a lot of weight, but he looks like himself. He'll look almost the same to you."

But something's happened to him between the time I saw him late in the afternoon and now, because when we walk into that room all the lights are off but the yellow light above his bed. He looks dead. They've propped up his bed, but his head has slipped off the pillow and it hangs to the side. There is no muscle tension in his face, no tautness, no sense of consciousness. My heart is in a panic. Maybe he really is dead.

"Dad?" I say. "Look who's here. I told you Carol was coming." He doesn't stir. I touch his arm, rub it a little, kiss his forehead. His skin is still warm, though a little papery. His face is smooth. We sit for a few minutes and wait. Suddenly I am inside the falling dream, and he's slipped through my frantic hands. I place my hand on his chest, feel the rise and fall of his breath. I turn my face away. Just a deep, deep sleep. I check the bladder bag, on which no one had painted a daffodil. It's about a fifth full of yellow brown liquid. So his kidneys are still working. But his great heart is slowing down.

"He didn't look like this a few hours ago," I whisper. "When I left him he didn't look like this," I say again. She just looks at me like I've lost my mind.

I check with the nurses' station. Just sleeping, they tell me, go on home. So I take my cousin to the house, put her to bed, sleep with the phone by my pillow. Well, he's just in a deep sleep. Actually he's on the edge of some other state, somewhere between deep sleep and coma I think. But he's still here. And he's in no pain. Or no pain that can speak from that far place he's gone to now.

Thursday he's come back to us. Carol walks into the room and his face lights up. "Oh!" he says with such surprise. Her red hair catches his eye right off. "You're *here*." He has forgotten she's coming and it makes a lovely surprise. It's the kind of surprise I wish I could conjure up every day, but our family is so small we've run out of surprises.

She's brought some photographs her father had taken during the war, when he was an air force photographer. She shows my father a picture of some general sitting in a jeep with FDR and asks if he knows who it is, and my father tells her right away. It's the last question my father is able to answer. These are her archives, her relics, pictures taken by her father, who has also died, and it brings him back to her a little to know this picture. We both have the sense that there are so many things that will never be known to us now, that we should have been more vigilant, asked more questions, written down more. All these stories of lives lived in shadow and light, arcs of life and death, secrets and longing, all lost.

I have a long talk with Jim, the night nurse, before I leave. He'd faxed my father's doctor two days ago for something called Oxyfast, for the last moments. But the doctor has left town for a long weekend without leaving orders for anything. Finally we contact his associate, who orders only a weak morphine drop they can put under my father's tongue. Jim's worried that it won't even come close to being strong enough, if it comes to that. I don't ask what that is exactly because such agony I can't hear about. The word *death rattle* rises up like a scrim of blackbirds across my sight and suddenly I can't see. I shut my eyes to close them out.

Jim wants me to sleep on the couch at the end of the hall. But this I cannot do. He tells me how he could not get to his mother before she died. There are tears in his eyes even now after all this time. That's why he's signed on for this tour of duty, so no one would die alone. I tell him I've made my peace with this, but I have not. "I can get here in twenty minutes," I say, "but I can't sleep here." I can barely sleep at home.

"I can't keep a vigil," I try to explain.

"You don't have brothers or sisters who can help you out? You could take turns."

"No," I say, "it's just me."

"Oh," he says, "I'm sorry. It's hard to do this alone."

"I have my husband and my children. But they have their lives, and I hate to ask too much."

So after I tell my father goodnight, I turn my back to the couch at the end of the hall and head on home. I tuck the phone against my pillow hoping it will never ever ring. Hours go by. The Oxyfast never comes.

It's Sunday and the sun is streaming in the windows. The mountains glisten in the sun from the early spring snow that fell during the night. I want to just stand there and look at the mountains and the water off in the distance, glinting now under the morning sun. It's an Easter kind of morning, though of course Easter was three weeks ago.

I'm there by myself to read my father the Twenty-third Psalm, tell him it's all right to let go. I want a little while alone with him to say goodbye before everybody else shows up. I know it's very close now, and I want to have a goodbye that's just mine with some ritual or ceremony. Suddenly I wish I were Buddhist, or Jewish, or Catholic. I wish I had incense and smoke, or chanting or song. My austere Methodist, then Presbyterian upbringing, has left me nothing to draw upon. Except for the Lord's Prayer I know no prayers I can say out loud. It occurs to me I could sing it to him right now better than I could say it. But I know my voice can't hold a tune. It can barely get through this reading.

I touch my father's arm, kiss his forehead. "Hi, Dad, it's me." His eyes are open and unblinking. The nurse says they're putting drops in them to keep them moist. It should be frightening to see him like that, but it's not. He's been like this since yesterday. I think he's holding on and letting go. But he can't stay like this forever. That this is the end both shocks and comforts me. The world should take such note. But of course it just rushes on through its doggy life, as the poet says, taking no notice whatsoever.

I pick up the Bible my minister grandfather had given him. I read the inscription again: "I'm so glad that you ever came to live with me." Suddenly I remember a letter my father wrote me when I was in college that ended with those very words. The child, the precious child, a gift from the universe. I read the Twenty-third Psalm without expression, almost in a whisper. I am self-conscious and just barely holding on to myself. Hospice workers have been reading this passage to him all week so my failure now doesn't strike me like it might.

The Lord is my shepherd. I shall not want. He maketh me to lie down in green pastures. He leadeth me beside the still waters. He restoreth my soul: he leadeth me in paths of righteousness for his name's sake. Yea, though I walk through the valley of the shadow of death, I will fear no evil: for thou art with me, thy rod and staff they comfort me. Thou preparest a table before me in the presence of mine enemies: thou anointest my head with oil; my cup runneth over. Surely goodness and mercy shall follow me all of the days of my life: and I will dwell in the house of the Lord for ever.

I want the comfort of those words but cannot find them. But to believe in such things—that one might have a companion for the walk through that dark valley. To be so loved and anointed with oil. My child, my child.

I get up and look at the water and the mountains again. I can believe in the beauty of the world, even as I stand by Lloyd's bed on the floor, his desk and computer, untouched since that night a week ago. Except for the bloodstains on the pillow, by all appearances he'll be coming back anytime now. But of course Lloyd isn't coming back at all. By now he's dead and gone, though no family has come to claim his things and make amends to the room. No hurry. The guy in the other bed is too busy checking out himself to notice any blood.

I turn and look at my still and silent father seeing the world for the last time. He's skimming on the top of a lifetime now. He's traveling so fast he can see everything. I hold on to his arm. Tell me all you can see is light, that there is no darkness anywhere. I touch his face. But where will you be when you are gone?

That afternoon we all meet in his room, where he is virtually lying in state.

We are not solemn, though I see flickers of our grief and fear pass among us, beneath our unguarded eyes. I thought then that we should have begun a vigil, a deathwatch, but instead we are taking my cousin out to dinner by the water, as she's leaving in the morning. We laugh at everything because tonight everything's funny. My mother sits gathered into herself, staring off at the water. It's all right. I'll go back after this dinner by the water to say goodnight, stay until I can't stay any longer. My mother passed the torch to me long ago. I feel it heavy in my hand.

That night my uncle comes to my daughter in a dream. She walks into the nursing home and there is her grandfather lying on the bottom bunk. He's dressed in white. Then she looks again and the bed is empty. But when she looks up she sees Uncle Henry in the top bunk wearing his yellow see-through shirt and brown wool jacket, his Scandinavian walking shoes. He's holding my father in his arms, and he's smiling that Uncle Henry smile. Who would have guessed it? My uncle as the go-between. And so my father had come on up at last. Who would have thought it? My doubting uncle as an angel.

Monday morning comes full of light. The April sun shines on, as it has shone all week. My daughter comes early. She's there to say goodbye, sit with him, touch him. Nothing can stop us from touching him now. He can't edge his arm away anymore. My husband brings my cousin to say goodbye, then takes her to the airport. My daughter goes to work, and I am alone. His eyes look out unblinking as they had since Friday. Nothing catches them now. Nothing makes them flicker. The nurse comes in with the eyedrops.

"Can I do this?"

"Yes. And you can do other things too."

I try to think of it as an anointing. I wipe his mouth and lips with a little sponge on a Q-tip, put two drops in each eye.

"He's still here," she says. "Talk to him. He can still hear you. Hearing is the last sense to go." She stands there, watching.

So I tell him it's all right now. We will be fine. We will take care of her forever, though of course I've said these things to him already. In Lisa's presence it's like a scene from a movie. I watch my words float up and break apart.

She takes his pulse, checks the bladder bag. He looks both dead and alive.

"How long can this go on?" I ask. This death fugue.

"We don't ever know exactly," she says. "Not long."

My mouth is dry, my heart is a knot in my throat. "I know it's the end," I say. "I really do." Suddenly I want to run away from this room, from his dying, so close now. "I think I need to eat something. Could I go have some lunch?"

"We have some yogurt in the fridge you could have. Or you could make a sandwich."

"I mean could I leave for just a little while?" My breath is coming fast now.

She tells me of course, though I see the way her eyes pull back from me. You should stay right here. You shouldn't move an inch. You haven't even slept on the couch. Then I hear my mother's voice: save yourself for the long haul. But of course there is no long haul. Yet an hour can be a long haul. And I was so hungry and shaky now and my husband was coming back to take me out for a little break. If I am to get through these last days or hours, I'll have to pace myself. Eat, drink, take deep breaths. Infidel that I am.

My growing terror finally gets me out of the nursing home. I practically run to the car. I open the window to that trickster April air, lean my head back, shut my eyes. "I won't be gone long," I say to no one in particular. In a house of death no more. Then I'm in that crowded lunchtime restaurant waiting for my bowl of soup. All these people. All these lives. I resent every one of them, their seeming happiness, their obliviousness. I hear a high note of laughter over the ticking of silverware, scraping of plates, footsteps, music in the background. Of course the anger is only for me. I'm the one who's gone AWOL.

"What if he dies while I'm gone?" I say to my husband.

"Is that why you left? It's okay, you know."

The tears I've been holding back all morning slide down my face unabashed. He brushes his hand across my cheek, my shoulders.

"If you're supposed to be there, you will be."

"But I shouldn't have left him."

"You need to eat something first. It won't be long now."

"I know. That's why I shouldn't have left."

"I meant the food," he says.

"I don't think I can eat anything after all." But in another moment our lunch arrives. It won't take long to gulp down this bowl of soup, this hot, creamy soup, which sets off my hunger with the first spoonful. Suddenly I could eat everything in the world. "It's good to do this," I say. "Can we just take our time then?"

But he knows me well enough not to trust this momentary reprieve. "We need the check now," he says, handing the server his credit card.

"You did a good job, you know," my husband says.

"So did you. You were so strong with him."

He shuts his eyes, shakes his head, then looks up at me. "I'm proud of you."

He drops me off and dashes back to work. He's only fifteen minutes away. "Call me if anything changes."

I rush into my father's room and sit down. "Hi, Dad. I got some lunch. I'm all right now." Nothing has changed. I have missed nothing. But I think how foolish it was to run off like that. A failure of nerve. Call it what you will, that's what it was.

Suddenly my father cries out though he can make no sound. His mouth opens wide and his eyes shut tight against some shuddering, silent pain. I do not look away. I resist the urge to run into the hall after the nurse. Maybe this is the death rattle if we could but hear it. A great washing over of pain as the body says goodbye to earth. A cry for all he's leaving behind, his ambivalence to the end. Those morphine drops won't even come close to being strong enough, if it comes to that. Jim's words catch at my throat. So that's what the Oxyfast was for. I wait for it to happen again, but it doesn't. He goes back to the slow, shallow breathing as before. His eyes are open again and stare out across the room. Jim's on the night shift, so he's hours away. A little piano jazz right now would be nice. Lloyd rises from his bloody bed and floats across the room.

I have never told anyone this. My story has always been of his slow, easy death. But it was exactly like my uncle's soundless wail. A sound like that you tuck away and keep against all forgetting.

Soon his breathing changes—it's a little sandpapery now, whish, whish, and I go get the nurse. I'd forgotten for the moment that he can't be saved. Soon the hospice chaplain arrives. I have never met her before. So this is it, then. He is clearly losing his hold to earth now, and they have called her in for the finale. She tries to take my hand, but I slip it from her. I don't want to be touched either.

I scoot my chair as close to him as I can. The change is profound.

"Tell me about your father," she begins. "What are your favorite memories?"

I can't imagine such questions as comfort. I just look at her and turn back to him.

Finally I say, "The zoo. We liked the zoo."

"Tell me about that."

Go away! I want to scream, but polite to the end, I hold my tongue. They think I need company for this final stretch. They don't know I've been here already. They don't know how strong I've grown. I didn't know it myself until now. This is sacred space, and I want it all to myself. I have no need of interpreters now. Father Bill is all I need, and he's hidden safely inside. "We are not our bodies. We are not our minds. We are not our emotions, though they are all part of us. Our truest self is a spirit place that has always been there. He's going toward it now. Everything else is falling away."

I lay my cheek against my father's forehead. It's warm and dry. I want to see him slip from earth. I want to see where he's going. We don't need words anymore, do we. Ah, Dad, we really don't.

He's as still and quiet as anyone could possibly be. His eyes hold a fierce light.

They're looking out at something I can't see. They glisten from the eyedrops. And it's the drops, not tears, that trickle down his face. I take his face in my hands so that I'm not letting him go but taking him in.

His death, when it finally comes, is a choreography of grace. It is exactly like his brother's—the twin commas of breath between long, then longer rests, then finally the eyes closing slowly, as if on cue. My father never raged against the coming of the night or frayed into complaint. He went gently, with all his gentleness intact.

When my mother arrives with my husband, she takes one look at him and turns her face. "Would you like to touch him? Would you like to be alone with him?" I say.

No. No. She shakes her head. We circle the bed, hold hands. The hospice chaplain offers a prayer. I don't remember what. They give my mother his wedding ring, which slips easily off his finger. That night she slips it on a gold chain she wears around her neck.

My father's face is slack, but his color abides. He looks to be in a deep sleep even now, half an hour later, as though part of him still has not completely let go. I want to feel his spirit hover over us, looking down. Come back, I say to my secret heart. I want him to be someplace and not just gone. His body is not a shell, though my mother will not touch him.

Then my husband takes my mother home to their University House apartment—to my father's clothes and his books and all the things that would not fit into his little half room at the nursing home. All the things she could not get rid of though she knew he was never coming back.

House of Widows

My mother is the newest widow in the House of Widows. I hoped many things for her in this, the worst and best part of her old age. She was never really able to make close friends at University House during the time my father was alive, and now I hoped she would. If not the slumber parties in the girls' dorm like I'd imagined when she came here, at least coffee and cookies in the afternoon, or wine and cheese before dinner, and then, a little University House gossip in one apartment or another into the evening.

But this is no college dorm. There are gentle signs of affection, little cards and notes left on the ledges outside doors, a phone call now and then for a dinner date, an occasional lunch. But everything is tentative now, and there is too much risk in fierce attachments. I watch women walk down the hall together after dinner, each turning at her own door. No invitation to come in, sit a spell, gossip a little, share secrets, laugh. These solitary women lead private lives behind their doors. And maybe after a lifetime of attachments and service to others, solitude now might feel cool and lovely, a thing apart.

I wonder what they do behind their closed doors in their dreaming lives. After all, how long would it take to trace the edges of your life—how long to feel the contours of your soul, to sink deeply into the dark rivers of memory and desire? Ah, such days for smoothing out the sorrows and regrets of life. Who can tell how much of life remains at eighty or even ninety to be held tenderly in such trembling hands? Once I had thought I would like to interview women who had reached this age, but then shrank from it. *Don't patronize me with your notebook or tape recorder asking me about my life. My life is not yours for the asking.* And of course what I seek both then and now is reassurance. *It's not so bad as it seems. See? Here in my hands are the riches of my old age. I am here to tell you of the contentment of that dark river I drift in.* But I was not ready to hear of the ravages and insults of old age. I could not bear this then, not the details of that road awaiting us all.

And so I began to imagine the comforts of sex in the dark in this House of Widows. I wondered how these women managed it. If, when they moved in as widows, they came with a double bed—or if they'd downsized to a single to make room for the large dresser and the comfortable bedroom chair. I wished them much sex in the dark. No need for sight now. Candlelight might be nice. Touch would be all you needed. Any woman would be lovely in a pale-green, shimmery nightgown and robe. Her face would be radiant when her elderly lover's practiced if unsteady hands slid over the landscape of her body, first here and there, tentative but full of wonder and surprise that everything was as it has always been. Hands and mouths would do just fine. No need for everything you once had to be in tiptop working order. Love among the elderly should never be a joke. We should never grow too old for that.

My mother had stopped wearing makeup the day of my father's stroke. And as weeks and months, then years, wore on, I believe she forgot the pleasure in the ritual, the transformation. She was always beautiful to me, and beautiful without any touchups here and there. But it was an effacement so absolute, it frightened me. So I hoped that one day she would look in the mirror and say, *Okay, world, here I am,* and wish for a little lipstick, a little blush. Sometimes when I look in the mirror at night I see my mother's face looking back instead of my own, and I think of her life alone, and it's the saddest thing in the world. There are many such sorrows.

Then one day, a few months after my father died, my mother announces that she's ready for a change. "I want an extreme makeover," she tells me. "Take me to Nordstrom. Let's go have the works." I set up an appointment and off we go. I can't wait. Eyeliner, eye shadow, eyebrow pencil, blush, foundation, lipstick. She buys it all. Then we go upstairs and buy a new red coat. It's her coming out and the first of many such transformations. The outward sign of an inner letting go, or taking hold.

After years in the shadow of my Republican father, my mother becomes a Democrat, and votes for John Kerry in her first Democratic precinct caucus. She becomes floor representative to the University House council, parliamentarian for the University House Association meetings. She gives coffee hour talks on her life. She buys season tickets to the symphony. She goes to the concerts held a couple of times a week in the University House auditorium. The music can move her to tears or offend her musical sensibility in a gentle, indulgent way. We buy her a CD player and some CDs to go with it: Gershwin, Corelli, Copeland, Mozart, Ravel.

Ed and I take her to dinner every Sunday night, keeping the traditions. My daughter and I take her to movies. I take her to lunch. Sometimes I swing by after work and take her to dinner. But she does not join the French club or the Shakespeare club or the book club or the current affairs discussion group or the bridge club or even the Red Hat Society. She tries the Grieving Widows club once, but gives it up after the first meeting. Too depressing. "I just like to read," she says, when I try to encourage some of these attachments. But she was never a joiner and neither am I. But read she does. Book after book after book from the well-stocked University House library, or from my own. She reads all 957 pages of Bill Clinton's autobiography, and she is the only person I know who has read all of the *9/11 Commission Report*.

Now that my father is gone, and there is no one who loves her best, or asks after her day, I make sure to call her every night no matter where I am. She keeps a little list during the day, in preparation for my call, putting down little gossipy anecdotes, and anything she thinks is interesting or funny. I love it. I love the comfort of hearing about the shape of her day and her happiness in it. There is almost always something strange and startling, in between the descriptions of what she had for dinner and who she ate it with.

"Well, I had a new experience, today," she says, in her usual understated way. She'd gotten a brochure in the mail from the Whitworth Alumni Association for the Whitworth College Choir tour schedule of appearances, with a number to call.

"So I called it," she tells me. "And you know what?"

I have no idea.

"Well, all I can say is that it was a very unfortunate misprint. Because I certainly didn't get the Whitworth Alumni Association."

"What? What did you get?"

"Oh I'd better tell you. You'll never guess." She's teasing me, stretching it out, waiting upon her own comic timing. "It was a sex talk hotline."

"What did you say?"

"I asked them what they could do for an eighty-eight-year-old widow."

Or her dreams. "Last night I dreamed I had a *torrid* affair with Alan Alda and left your father to run off with him. I just told you this to let you know I'm still alive." She loves Bill Clinton, also, and wrote him a fan letter that began "Dear Bill." But she hates George Bush so much that we had to make a phone call rule about it: we could not mention his name after nine o'clock at night.

My mother keeps a prayer list beside her bed, next to my father's leather-bound New Testament, and a booklet of devotional readings. And after me, my husband, and our three kids, number six on her prayer list is George W. Bush. Though she hates him, hates seeing his "beady little eyes," or hearing his voice on television, or his name in casual conversation, when my mother says her prayers, she says a prayer for George W. too.

My mother and I have a ritual at night that quiets my fast-beating heart and tells me that all is well as we sink into our little incantation of comfort.

"Are you wearing your cozy robe?" I ask. I had bought her a white, plush chenille robe, which she loves more than anything I've ever given her.

"Well, are you in your cozy pajamas?" she says back. "Have you taken off your bra? You can't be relaxed until you do that."

"I love my solitude," my mother tells me often. I do everything I can to believe her, and mostly I do. But sometimes when I make my nightly check-in call, her voice goes soft and she says, "I've been reading your father's book." I know what she means. She's living in my father's words and her part in them. *The Presidents' Last Years*. On the back of her chair, when she isn't wearing it herself, she keeps his favorite beige sweater, the one that always washed him out. And then I think how she must be missing his company in the other TV chair, watching the late-night news as was their custom. So now she lets the news put her to sleep. Stories of murders and fires and other disasters don't touch her. She lets the comfort of voices ease her into sleep, along with the one who is both as close as breathing and gone too far for breath.

Six months after my father's death, Bill Stylstra dies. Ann Stylstra helped Bill ease his way out of life one long night, across the hall from my mother. My mother begins to refer to Ann by her proper name. *Angelyn*, she says with a kind of whispery reverence. *Angelyn*. I had never heard her use this name before. But I know what it is. My mother is acknowledging the sacred space her friend from across the hall has entered, that shimmering place where one is kept safe from despair by the tugs and pulls from both the living and the dead, where the beloved dead are always a full moon at noontide.

Then Buffy Parsons, in her nineties, who had lived in Africa with her doctor husband, Bill. He died hours after he'd carried the lead in a Readers Theater production. They had invited friends in to celebrate with wine and cheese and toasts to his long life, and then in the night he died. And finally, Anne Raymond. I remember how she turned to Hank as they came down the hall one day, and gave him such a smile it was as if their lives would go on forever, as if they still made love every day to prove it. A few weeks later, they rushed Hank to the hospital, then took him to a convalescence center, where he lingered for months, before Anne joined the ranks of the other widows of the third floor.

When my father was alive, my mother used to refer to having dinner with *The Stylstras, The Raymonds, The Parsons.* As she herself was once part of *The Cunninghams.* Now she is simply, wholly herself. *Grace.* Now there are other couples she joins—*The Halls* or *The Goodes*, making it a threesome, or if another joins them, a foursome. But she doesn't admit to envy or even recognition of this linguistic sleight of hand that gives women back to themselves both more and less.

Ginny becomes my mother's best friend, a friend who takes the place of my father sometimes during that dark hour before dinner and for a little while after. Once Ginny and my mother planned a little conspiratorial soiree to rescue a man new to The House from the clutches of a man-hungry woman named Susan, who had gathered him up before he could take off his hat and coat. Ginny and my mother invited him over for wine and cheese, then took him to dinner, just to show Susan, and I suppose each other, that she wasn't the only woman who could still have some fun with a man. But Susan got him anyway. Ginny and my mother made jokes that she'd somehow magnetized or Velcroed him, because she got him never to leave her side. Of course, neither my mother nor Ginny is interested in actually *having* boyfriends themselves. They're done with all that. But it was great fun, and Ginny was a kindred spirit with my school administrator mother, who loved skinny-dipping, tap dancing, and anything that was both safe and forbidden. My mother believed in a woman's right to abortion and to her own life long before *Roe v. Wade.* She believed in me and in whatever shape my life might take. But she had been tamped down so long by my father's illness that this breaking free with Ginny, just for a season, before Ginny became too ill, was lovely to see.

Later, Ginny fell in the night and got wedged in between the bed and the wall and lay there for hours before someone found her. "I can't go anywhere in this old thing," she'd said of her nightgown, when the medics finally arrived to take her to the hospital. So at her direction, the two medics helped her out of her old one and into a new, pretty one before they carried her out on the stretcher. But Ginny battled back, and finally returned to University House, where she led a diminished, anxious life, until she died. Ginny was my mother's first and best friend at University House, whom she mourned for many months, until even Ginny faded into a backdrop of faces come and gone.

Now I walk by Apartment 320 every time I visit my mother, who has moved to a single-bedroom apartment down the hall. I always pause and look at the new name over the door and feel such sadness wash over me. Sometimes I stop and touch the door for the briefest of seconds. That's the last place my parents were together, the last place before their life together came to an end. It's where I would wish to go now and sit and just look at them and never mind the smell at all. I could just sit on the couch and it wouldn't matter if they fell asleep as soon as the flush of my entrance had worn off and my mother would say, "Homer, you're sleeping! Ann's here." I wouldn't even have to touch them. To see them again outside of dreams would be enough.

I had the falling dreams on and off for several years after my uncle and my father died, though I don't have them anymore, even though my mother has fallen several times in recent months. She tripped over her walker and fell and hit the side of her face on the chest in the hall of her apartment. She bruised her face terribly, but it could have been much worse. She could have smacked the back of her head or her temple, and she could have hemorrhaged. She's on Coumadin at the moment for a blood clot in her calf, which had put her in the hospital for a week, a couple of months ago, and which probably also had sent a little showering of clots to her brain, marking the beginning of the many ways she will fall.

It's a Friday, and Ed has a basketball game, so I call my mother from school to arrange a dinner date. "I'll swing by after work," I tell her. "We can go to the Rusty Pelican and split the chocolate brownie for dessert."

"Oh, I would love that," she says, since this is her next-to-favorite restaurant and her next-to-favorite dessert. "Do you want me to be downstairs in the lobby, or do you want to come up?"

I tell her I'll come to her apartment. "You never know how Friday traffic's going to be, but I should be there about four thirty."

I'm there right on the money. Four thirty. Traffic was easy and I'm getting hungry. And today for some reason I especially need to see her. I knock twice and let myself in.

"Mom? Hey. I'm here."

But she's not in the bathroom or the bedroom or the living room. She's nowhere. Of course, I think she's fallen again and they've taken her away in an ambulance. I rush down three flights of stairs to the Wellness Center. If anything has happened to her, they would know.

"Your mom? Oh she was just here getting her blood pressure reading. She's gone off to dinner." This is almost as frightening as the ambulance. I make my way down the long hall to the dining room. I stand in the doorway and see my mother at at a table of lively women, as she sits with her head down, slowly putting the fork to her mouth. When had she grown so quiet? I slip away and go to the car and put my head on the steering wheel, and cry. Here we are, I think. Here we are.

But she's so smart, and she has compensated so well for so long, the extent of her brain loss is not clear to any of us for quite a while.

"Anything you want to bring up?" I ask her on our way to the medical appointment where the doctor will give her the findings of the MRI taken of her brain, which I already know.

"No, I don't think so. I think I'm doing pretty well."

Sure, Ma, you bet. It's the only answer there is.

The doctor asks if she has any trouble remembering things.

"No, I don't think so. Do I, Ann?"

"Well, yeah, Mom, sometimes you do." She looks at me sharply. It is a betrayal. The doctor gently suggests that she might need to be in a place that is safer for her, where she would get better care.

It's the wrong choice of words. "But I have *wonderful* care."

"Well. Down the line, Grace. When you may need a little more help than you do now. It might be better to find a different place now rather than later."

"'But I'm managing just *fine*."

On the ride home she is completely silent. "Mom, what are you thinking?"

"That I can't stand Dr. Mitchell."

"Why?"

"He's so *obsequious*."

I laugh. For a moment a flush of relief washes over me. Anybody who can use the word *obsequious* in casual conversation could not have a shrinking brain.

Then she goes silent again. So I ask what she took from the visit.

"That I'll have to move and it makes me sad." The last place where she and my father were together. All the grooves and nooks and crannies, the smells and rhythms, the color, the music, all that light. Goodbye to everything.

"It wouldn't be a nursing home, Mom. Just an assisted living place where they can look out for you a little more."

And so we move her from University House to an assisted living community called Crista, which gives her three meals a day instead of one, and whatever help she needs along the way. And now our house is only fifteen minutes away.

We've downsized her from a three-room apartment, to a single room with just her bed, which we put next to the window, her little table for eating snacks and putting on her makeup, her easy chair, a chair for a guest, a small bookshelf, her TV, and a refrigerator. She shares a bathroom with the woman next door, who is the shortest woman I have ever seen. Since my mother needs a booster seat on the toilet to get up and down, they must bring in a stepping stool for my mother's tiny neighbor.

I've bought my mother new linens and a new bedspread, new towels, some artificial flowers, everything I can think of to make it lovely for her. Ed tucks the oxygen tank as discreetly as he can behind her chair in the corner, where it hisses and thumps all day and all night. It's attached to my mother's cannula by fifty feet of tubing that snakes after her wherever she goes, though unbelievably it never trips her up. No glass sculptures or elegant reading room with a grand piano here, but it's cozy and warm and the attendants and nurses are wonderful to her, though she can't remember their names. Crista has an adjacent nursing home, which is where she will probably end up, and it's lovely too, as those things go. There are parakeets in little cages in the hallways, something I put much faith in when I first looked at this place.

My mother has long ago stopped making lists for our nightly phone call, then later stopped remembering that I called at all. I can't ask after her day, or what she had for dinner or what was in the news, since she can't remember that far back and she has stopped watching TV altogether. So I launch into my little mono- logue of things that would interest her, trying to be funny enough over the phone for both of us.

"Ma? Are you there?"

"I'm here," she says with a start, and I know I've wakened her.

That's what the call is all about anyway. It's a litany of mother-daughter love, each saying to the other, *I'm here. I won't leave you. I won't go away in the night.*

And my visits are different now. After an hour or so my monologue wears thin and she's drifting in and out of sleep, sitting reclined in her chair, her eyes closed.

But as I get up to leave, she says, "I love it when you come. I just like to hear you talk." And I sit back down. When I finally do leave, I rush out of there, glad to be free of that place and my mother's raspy breath, which is her death in her, and the hiss and thump of the oxygen tank. I cry all the way home. I haven't stayed long enough or come often enough no matter how long I stay or how often I come.

We still take her out for our Sunday night dinner ritual, and the staff gets her all gussied up for her night out on the town. Sometimes when we bring her home from dinner she heads off to the bathroom, then comes out a few minutes later and asks, "Where should I go now?"

At first I don't know what she means. It's a one-room apartment. Where else is there to go but her chair, unless she wants to go to bed, and it's way too early for that.

"Where do you want to go?" I say.

She gives me a long look that I cannot read and says finally, "My chair."

Later I realize that she's asked because she can't remember whether we've just been to dinner or are just getting ready to go to dinner. It's all right. That lapse is forgotten in a moment too.

So many things best unremembered. These failures of the body, one by one, and now the mind—this most surprising failure of all. But this unremembering is a gift that even in my grief I recognize. I am thinking now of my husband cleaning up my dignified mother after she had soiled herself that last winter when she was so ill. This had never happened to her before in her life. So now it has come down to this, even for her, whom I have promised to leave out of this story. Yet as excruciating as it must have been for her and for him, those secrets of the body forever link us to each other and inscribe our lives upon Hawthorne's "magnetic chain of humanity." And they tell us how little that kind of dignity matters when what matters most is love.

It's four years after my father's death, and Christmas Eve, my mother's very last, and we all know it. The staff has gotten her dressed up in her black wool pantsuit and red coat for our holiday dinner at Scott's Grill. We all wear Christmas tree pins that blink on and off. My mother orders a margarita before dinner. We have a grand toast to the holiday, then my mother orders cod with sour cream for her entrée and her favorite, chocolate soufflé, for dessert. She laughs, makes a great joke that I cannot remember. On Christmas Day at our house she's quiet, has trouble opening her presents, or remembering who to thank. That night on the way back to her apartment, as we walk into the foyer at Crista, she says she's going to be sick. I grab my wool scarf and she throws up in it.

"I'm so sorry," she says. Ed and I get her inside. We stay with her a little while. I bring her some cold water, touch her face. The attendant comes in to get her ready for bed, give her her night pills. I put the new Christmas clothes I've bought her in her closet. Put her other presents away.

"I feel better now. You'd better go on home."

We kiss her goodnight.

When the phone rings the next morning, I have no feeling of foreboding or dread. "We called an ambulance for your mother," Marilee, the head nurse, tells me. "She seemed disoriented this morning and had trouble standing up. They're taking her to Northwest Hospital."

My husband and I rush after her, meet her in the ER. It's pneumonia come out of nowhere. Except that my mother's been on oxygen since September, and that raspy catch in her chest has only gotten worse. She's in the hospital four days.

After my father died she took to studying the obituaries in the paper. "When I read that someone died after a short illness, I think how lucky that person is. I'd be grateful for those words after my name." I know she's thinking of how long my father took to die.

So when I come to the hospital in the morning of the third day and learn from the charge nurse that the pneumonia is now in both lungs, that the antibiotics are doing nothing to stop it, I know immediately what she would want me to do. When I go into her room, I see she's watching Gerald Ford's funeral. She has a special interest in this, of course, because my father had met him and they had that fine picture taken together.

"How are you, Mom?" I say, touching her arm.

"I had a hard night," she says. "I think I had a bad reaction to some medication. But I'm much better systemically."

I sit awhile and watch the ceremony, then go out into the waiting area to call my cousin, Carol. She should know how things are. When I come back, my mother is struggling to get out of bed and saying she has to get to dinner.

I dash into the hall and call for the nurse. "Something's happening to my mother!" Two nurses rush in and check her oxygen saturation levels. I can see for myself what they are: 76. They clamp on an oxygen mask and turn up the pressure as high as it can go. Even so, she's delirious and in and out of some other reality. "We were just talking about Gerald Ford," I say, as if I can hardly believe what is happening.

When I can step outside the room I find my mother's nurse and ask, "What does 76 mean? It sounds pretty low."

"It means not compatible with life."

They want to put her in the ICU. *Comfort care,* I say, only comfort care now. No rushing to the ICU. Only warm and soft and easy as you go. After a brief illness. I know now that she will get her wish.

This time I'm not alone. My husband and my cousin, Carol, and her husband are here, having flown up from California on a moment's notice. We circle the bed, touch her everywhere, play Mozart, dim the lights. The kids have come and gone. Each one in turn has said a private goodbye. Just after midnight, my practical, no-nonsense mother dies.

I watch her spirit leave her body within moments, watch her face change into a death mask before me and become someone else. It's all right. She'd wanted to be out of her body for so long—no ambivalence here, not a moment wasted going where she wants to go.

Come on up, the twins say. It's great up here. My father reaches down to give her a lift.

The Long Shadows of Winter

The summer after my father died, when I still had a mother, I waited for a sign from him. I had not thought to ask him for that. The pair of bluebirds, ravishing in the sun, or the robins who'd made their nest in the rhododendron bush beside the garage, or the flickers, who lived under the eaves, or the owl that called from the woods as I'd stepped outside to say goodnight to the moon. Birds flushed out of the trees, a cry of annunciation or alarm. But which? Never before such a season of birds. Where are you? I said in the fall. The robin's nest abandoned, the bluebirds flown south in the failing light, the leaves floating through pale and gold-spun air, the woods absent of sound. Send me a sign that you are somewhere.

That same summer Alex died. She'd had a series of little strokes, and eventually couldn't walk, or even sit up, and no way to get outside. She lay on a blanket and pillow we'd spread for her in the kitchen in such despair we could not bear it. Just before we took her to the vet for the last goodbye, I remembered what I'd not thought to ask my father: "Stick around for a little while after you go," I said to her, "so I'll know you're still somewhere." And the next night, two thousand miles away, in Key West for a conference, I was almost asleep when I heard her breathing. I thought there was someone in the room, turned on the lights, but no one was there. The same thing happened the next night. I got up, thinking maybe it was the hair dryer in the bathroom, but everything remained as it was. Alex, I said. Then I settled back into sleep, into that warm, gentle sound of dog breath.

• • •

It's the middle of the night that first Thanksgiving without my father. My husband collapses in the bathroom. I am pulled out of sleep by three thumps or bangs my husband says he never made. I fly out of bed into the bathroom. I find him passed out on the floor. He looks dead. It isn't him, I think, because this is only a dream.

I don't see them take Ed out on the stretcher through the downstairs sliding glass door. I have not said goodbye or touched him, or whispered intimacies or kissed his face. I don't remember anything but the conversation with the medic about the dog, who's curious about all the commotion, but not alarmed. Are you all right? Alex says with her eyes. I watch the red taillights of the ambulance fishtail their way down the hill.

In my mind's eye I can see my mother on those trips she'd made to the ER with my father, sitting sideways on the seat in the back of the ambulance, touching my father's face or his wrist with her cold, cold hand, or sitting in the front next to the driver making small talk over the siren gone silent because there is no traffic and the roads are bare. Me, I throw on a coat and rush after the ambulance into the fog. I lost them after the first turn.

But here I am in my pajamas underneath my jeans and yellow sweatshirt. They've sent me out to the waiting room while they do something to my husband I shouldn't see. It's four in the morning, the hour of the wolf, and the only light in the room is from the Christmas tree in the corner. I am alone. I am more alone than I have ever been. And it's all too achingly familiar. All those trips to the ER with my father rise up before me. The sound of soft shoes up and down the linoleum hallway, the cannula in the nose, the hiss and sputter of the blood pressure machine, the heart monitor, the nitro, the works, as it was all those times before.

I'm looking at the Christmas tree and trying not to cry. The elevator slides up and the doors open, but nobody's there. The first time it happens it startles me, but I've been here so long now I hardly notice it. I hear the *ka thunk* and there it is again. But this time, I look up, and when the doors open, there he is. My father walks out of the elevator and steps toward me. He steps out of the lighted square of the elevator and looks around until he sees me. He doesn't say anything at all. He was never calm in emergencies but he's calm now. He's wearing his Dockers and a beige shirt and his beige sweater. No words of advice, no look into the future, no invitation to the other side.

It's all right, Pill, it's all right. He's light now. His steps are steady and light. He's not bound by anything but the pulls and tugs of earthly love. Oh to have lost you, never to see your face again on this earth. I could not bear it, he said. It only lasts a second or two. I shut my eyes to keep him there. But I have seen his face. Now I have seen his face. And the long wait through the loss of him is over.

I sit for a long time, staring at the elevator. Every so often it rises and the doors open to an empty square of light. I shut my eyes and will it to happen again, then realize I'd never willed it to begin with. I don't know how long I've been sitting in this room and suddenly the thought frightens me. Then the old terror rises up from years ago, and I'm back in that hospital room watching it snow, waiting for my husband's cancer surgeon to come back with the report.

But there's no snow here in this season of waiting, just cold and fog. The windows show me my own frantic reflection, which I don't immediately recognize. Then I'm rushing down the long hall, lit up like any other day, and almost collide with the nurse turning into my husband's room.

"It's not cancer, is it?" I whisper fiercely to the nurse, who appears to be backing away from me as fast as she can. "There's no way this could be cancer. Could it?"

I've startled her with my terror, and she just looks at me and shakes her head. "I don't know," she says more gently than I deserve. "We're only checking his heart." She takes my arm. She's probably used to the hysterics of wives who wait.

But I can't let her go. I ask her questions she can't possibly answer.

Finally she says, "Just go in and sit by him. It's best to do that right now."

"You're turning into your mother," my husband says when I come into the room. He's not nearly as groggy as he should be and has heard everything.

"God, I hope not," I say, but add, "at least she wasn't hysterical like me."

"I didn't mean that. I meant I'm not your dad. You don't have to hover like that."

"I know," I say. Then I sit down and whisper, "I saw him. I saw him coming out of the elevator." He knows exactly who I mean.

"Really?" he says.

"You believe me, don't you?"

"Of course."

"I knew you would. I shouldn't talk about it anymore." It's too attenuated to hold to the light, even in this room so strangely, softly lit. I ease down into the chair, put my head back, let out the breath I'd been holding these last few hours. Something has been settled. "I should call the kids."

"Let them sleep," my husband says. "What can they do?"

"Be here."

I lean over and touch his bare arm. It's warm and strong. I run my hand across his chest, put my palm over his heart through the thin hospital gown, feel the steady, slow pulse. My hand is not offended by the monitors sticking to him, tethering him to this other world. "You're warm," I say. Even in this unearthly light I can see that his color is good, as they say. His golden skin. I can't stop looking at his face. He's drifted back to sleep, but there is none of that terrifying slackness of before. Just the ease and comfort of pure sleep.

I look at the sun coming up over the edge of the rooftop, laying a rush of light across the gravel glittering in the sun. The air outside is cold and the sky is washed clean. I've only been in this twilight world for five hours, but I've already forgotten the sun. Now here it is after all.

"You called out to me," I say when he wakes up. "I heard you from my sleep."

"What do you mean?" he says. He has no recollection of those three thumps on the wall. I could hear them still.

That filament spun from his heart to mine had tugged and pulled, touching heart to heart. Well, heart was the subject at hand. He wasn't on the cardiac floor for nothing. Cancer had faded into the distance, for now, at least.

"Will our lives change then?" I ask. "I mean in what's coming."

"I don't know. Maybe. Probably not."

"How can they not? This terrible thing has happened again."

"We don't know that. Maybe nothing's happened."

"But I saw you dead."

"Come here," he says. And so I do. I edge onto the side of that narrow bed, put my face against his face.

Later that morning I run home to grab my husband's wallet, his insurance cards, reading glasses, feed the dog. I put the key in the lock like it's any old day. There's the dog, looking at me through the window by the door. I turn the key and step into an unearthly quiet. Even the dog is still. The winter sun fills the house with a vacant light. Now I know what it feels like to be a widow.

Well where is he? she asks me with her eyes, like she'd done with my father long ago. Where did you take him? She sniffs the hem of my jacket, noses my pockets, licks my hand. I sit down on the floor and bring her to me, hug her wide neck. She lets me stay like this for as long as I need to.

I find my husband's wallet in his pants on the floor, pull out the insurance cards. The house as we had left it. The unmade bed, the covers in a tangle. The candle we'd burned before we'd finally fallen asleep. In my mind's eye I watch my mother walk into their apartment to my father's socks and shoes and his sport coats, his winter hat and muffler, his handkerchiefs, the smell of him everywhere, his soft, lovely smell. She lies on the bed with her face in the pillow so no one can hear her cry.

Then I'm back at the hospital, walking through the waiting room of the cardiac unit where I'd spent the night. The Christmas tree in the corner winks and nods as I walk by. I lean over and breathe in the smell of Christmas. The sun is on everything. Out the window the city goes on as far as you can see. I look back at the elevator where my father had been, and make my way down the hall. I hear my husband's laugh as I round the corner. There are the kids, circling his bed. Somebody's said something funny and now everybody's laughing. The curtains are opened all the way, and the sun is pouring in. I stand in the doorway to his room, watching.

As it turns out, the heart attack was no heart attack at all, just the universe giving us a good shake. Death was not around some corner after all. Tomorrow would be just another day, like many other such days. There was no end to them. One way or another, we would outlive this all, even as we kept watch on the long shadows of winter.

Epilogue

Writing this now in a rainy light after loss upon loss, a memory comes to me. When I was a teenager, I took voice lessons from Ruth Havstad Almandinger, who gave me exercises and songs I hardly ever practiced. I have wondered why this memory has so suddenly come to me now, and why this, the only song I remember, comes back to me whole and complete:

> Oh! my lover is a fisherman
> > and sails on the bright blue river
> In his little boat with the crimson sail
> > sets he out on the dawn each morning
> With his net so strong
> > he fishes all the day long
> And many are the fish he gathers
> Oh! My lover is a fisherman
> And he'll come for me very *soon*!

If only I'd known then that my true love would be a fisherman, I might have practiced that song harder and sung it with more feeling, which was what Ruth Havstad Almandinger was always trying to get me to do. If only I'd had a grown-up glimpse of my true love when I was sixteen, I would have sung that song so well. If only I'd known he would have cancer and go to the lake for healing the summer after the radiation treatments were done. If only I'd known that I would be his fishing partner that miracle summer the sockeye came into the lake from the sea. If only I'd known that the cancer would return and that I would do everything I could to save him, knowing all along that he could not be saved, and that my heart would break beyond breaking, then break again. If only I'd seen the sun coming up over the mountains and the sky shift from gray to purple and the pale smudge of light against the mountains turn gold just above the crest. If only I'd seen the sun glinting off those sunslept waters as my love lets down the fishing lines, and off in the distance a salmon leaps—a silver flashing in the sky as if to split the heart of the sun—before it disappears into a soundless splash, in this all too brief and luminous season, to spawn and to die—oh, how I would have sung that song.

Acknowledgments

This book would not have come into being were it not for the abiding presence of the following people: Kathryn Lang, my editor at SMU Press, whose fierce and tender editing suggestions pushed me farther than ever I thought I could go; Bob Fullilove, who provided graceful and acute copyediting; Kristen Bergsman, whose early suggestions helped to ground the book in time and place; Lawrence Juhlin, family archivist, who uncovered the history of my grandmother Alfreda Juhlin; Julie Dinsmore, LiCSW, for her guidance and insight in all things big and small; Terry Conner, poet, fisherman, and friend; Mary and Phil Hickey, safe ports in any storm; Carol and Dick Zahniser, cousins whose gifts are laughter and love; Beverly Conner and Beth Kalikoff, writing group members and friends of my heart; Bonnie Tidball, my almost mother; Joan Becker, my almost sister, and her husband, Jim; Walter Hudsick and Phil Strable, who prove there are many ways to be a family; sister-in-law Theresa Stone and her husband Bill; Maureen Putnam, daughter-in-law extraordinaire; my children, Christopher, Robb, and Courtney Putnam, who live inside these pages and in my heart; and my grandbaby, Nicholas Christopher Putnam, for whom this book is both love letter and record. And finally, gratitude for my life with the threesome—my uncle, Henry Cunningham, and my parents, Homer and Grace Cunningham.

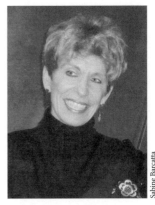

Sabine Barcatta

Ann Putnam teaches creative writing and gender studies at the University of Puget Sound in Tacoma, Washington. She has published short fiction, personal essays, literary criticism, and book reviews in various anthologies such as *Hemingway and Women: Female Critics and the Female Voice*, and in journals, including the *Hemingway Review*, *Western American Literature*, and the *South Dakota Review*.